LIVING THE STEPS TO VIBRANCY

Living The Steps to Vibrancy

AN *Intensive* PATH TO WHOLENESS
AND THE LIFE YOU OUGHT TO BE LIVING

RICHARD J. SANDORE, M.D.

Rikuys Press

LIVING THE STEPS TO VIBRANCY:
An Intensive Path to Wholeness and the Life You Ought to Be Living.
Copyright © 1999 by Richard J. Sandore, M.D.

First paperback edition published 1999

ISBN 0-9671522-1-6

Library of Congress Catalog Card Number: 99-90267

Published by
Rikuys Press
Box 540
Wadsworth, Illinois 60083
847-599-1885

Rikuys is a word in Quechua, an ancient language of the Andes, which means *visions.*

If you are unable to obtain this book from your local bookseller, you may order directly from the publisher by calling 1-888-97SPIRIT. Quantity discounts may apply.

Printed on acid free paper in the United States.

For

The little red fox who taught me so much
in a single, eternal morning,

and,

Karen, for selflessly taking care of me,
and allowing me to be me.

ACKNOWLEDGMENTS

Until you decide to write and publish a book, you have no way of realizing the community of gracious, loving, and tolerant people needed to give birth to the project. A special thank you to Karen for selflessly taking care of me all these years, and to Ananya for making me believe that it matters. Much gratitude to April Wilson, my editor, and Barbara Johnson whose steady hand and patience created the beautiful, vibrant cover. Thank you to all of the people who reviewed the manuscript over and over and allowed the concepts to congeal into an understandable form. Much love and gratitude to Cindy without whom these concepts would never have gelled. Cindy, I still have the cocktail napkins. A warm and loving wish to Sia, a woman who I never met and who lived in her own vibrancy until her life ended much to soon, whose words say so very much in only four lines, and to her brother, for his permission to reprint her thoughts to honor her and help heal others. Thank you to all of the holders of copyrights for their gracious permissions to reprint their words, and to those who have chosen to endorse this project. And lastly, thank you to all of the wise sages and mentors who have graced my life with their presence and wisdom, and a most special thank you to Pops.

Relive me.
Realize my fear.

Touch the flower.
Begin to be renewed.

Sia

This is in the end the only kind of courage that is required of us: The courage to face the strangest, most unusual, most inexplicable experiences that can meet us.   The fact the people have in this sense been cowardly has done infinite harm to life; the experiences that are called "apparitions," the whole so-called "world of spirit," death, all these things that are so closely related to us, have through our daily defensiveness been so entirely eliminated from life that the senses with which we might have been able to grasp them have atrophied.

Rainer Maria Rilke

TABLE OF CONTENTS

Introduction

*The goal of the hero trip down to the jewel point is to
find those levels in the psyche that open, open, open,
and finally open to the mystery of your Self being
Buddha consciousness, or the Christ. That's the
journey.*

Joseph Campbell

THE LATE JOSEPH CAMPBELL, probably the premier
mythologist of the 20th century, was asked in one of
many interviews by Bill Moyers about the meaning of
life, and what people are searching for. Mr. Campbell answered Bill
Moyers in his usual understated, innocent, yet infinitely knowing
style. "People," he said, "aren't searching for the meaning of life.
No. People are searching for the experience of being alive." He

continued by explaining that there is no inherent meaning in life. We bring meaning to it.

During the past century, we in the United States, and the Western world as a whole, have experienced material prosperity unimagined only a hundred years ago. The eighties unquestionably epitomized the search for the experience of aliveness through material goods and possessions. And now, the eighties come and gone, we have the object of our search, and still we are empty inside. A French Playwright regarding the French Revolution wrote, "Isn't the irony precious: finally realizing the object of our desires is far more terrifying than the journey to them." We have achieved the object of our search, yet we are a Prozac society where five of the top ten prescribed drugs are antidepressants. We are at the peak of economic prosperity, yet there is an underlying uneasiness, an angst pervasive within our society. Why?

The psychologist Abraham Maslow coined the term self-actualization. Self-actualization means many things to many people, but at its heart it suggests balance. It means being in balance with ourselves, our communities, and our world. It means being on the path that is right for each of us as an individual. It means being on our own personal path, and nobody else's. Very few of us are truly walking our own personal paths, the path correct for us as an individual. We, as individuals in the West, have colluded with the consensual and have become self-materialized instead of self-actualized.

Maslow's premise, also seen in the world's great spiritual traditions, is that once our basic needs for food and shelter are met we naturally, as spiritual organisms, desire to explore who we are. This quest is explicitly evident in native traditions where the four big questions are: Who am I? Where did I come from? Why am I here? Where am I going? The truth of our innate longing and searching is

2

also evident in any Third World community. People in rural areas, living intimately with nature, trusting in nature to provide what they need, have a sense of themselves and their place in the grand scheme of things that we in the West cannot even conceptualize. These people have an inherent peacefulness that arises from a self-actualized state, not the frenetic uneasiness we in the Western world have derived from a self-materialized state.

About six years ago I had the fortune of traveling along the Peruvian Amazon. Our group journeyed along the Great River Sea in a three-tiered live aboard boat for two weeks. One afternoon, after we had docked for the night, a group of us went out exploring some of the smaller tributaries in a motorized launch. It was just before dark, the shadows were becoming long, and stillness blanketed the area as the transition from day to night creatures was occurring.

As we headed inland along a narrow tributary we passed a small canoe. An Indian, a native of the Amazon basin not beholden to or bound by the persuasions of country or nationality, his wife, and their companion dog were traveling the opposite direction. The three of them barely fit into the small canoe loaded with plantains and other jungle fruits the Pachamama, the Mother Earth, had provided for them. The bounty from their day of harvesting made the canoe decidedly top-heavy and I wondered why it didn't tip over. We waved to them. They smiled back, white teeth against sun scorched lips and bronzed skin, and waved to us. We continued on our journey, and they continued on theirs.

It was dark by the time we finished our exploration and learned the ins and outs of piranha fishing. A half-moon cast silver shadows that rippled along the black water and guided us back towards the main tributary and our home away from home. As the tributaries we were gliding over grew wider, a small hut raised on stilts became visible in the distance about 300 yards to our left. A flicker of orange light reached out to us through the openings left in the wooden walls to serve as windows. It was apparent that the two people and dog we had passed earlier lived there. It was also apparent that they knew something about themselves and their place in the universe which we didn't. They were living the experience we had all traveled thousands of miles from our homes and families searching for. Those two radiant people were living *within the self-actualized state*. They were living in communion and balance with the natural world–a way of *being* we, in our Western culture, have disowned and distanced ourselves from.

The real lesson, at least for me, wasn't completely apparent until a few days later when we reached Leticia, Colombia. Leticia is a city of approximately one million located on the Amazon in the *Tres Fronteras,* the area where Peru, Brazil, and Colombia meet. It was immediately apparent as we disembarked to spend the afternoon exploring Leticia that Leticia was no different from any large city, Third World, or First. The stench of poverty hung over the area just as the smell of aging fish lingered over the impromptu waterside market.

As we explored the city, what we call poverty surrounded us–beggars, children playing in mud made from sewer water, men searching through the trash for morsels of food, women selling themselves. Yet these people living off the remains of the city were in some ways not so different from the couple living in the jungle. Both would be considered impoverished by our Western standards. Neither of them had the things, the goods and material possessions we desire so fiercely, and cherish and cling to so tightly. However, you could hardly call the couple living in their hut situated on the Amazon River impoverished or poor. Their very essence gently floated within the realm of harmony and balance so sorely lacking in the confines of Leticia.

Poverty, I came to realize, is a condition we have created for ourselves. It stems from being out of balance with ourselves, with our nature, and with our world. Poverty arises out of deviating from the longing within ourselves to see, to understand, to experience our true nature. It stems from stepping away from the quest for self-actualization. It arises from a condition of imbalance and disequilibrium. According to Maslow, materialism has led us astray from our true search, our true journey, and we are now just beginning to realize this. We have our material desires, and there is nothing inherently wrong with this, but we are recognizing that the material possessions are not what we need, they are not the end of our journey. We are realizing that our own search needs to begin within rather than outside of ourselves, and that until we address the four big questions: Who am I? Where did I come from? Why am I here? Where am I going?, we will not find the peace, balance, and harmony which we are missing, and so relentlessly seeking.

My own path and searching began just after I completed my medical training. I was in a lucrative private medical practice and working seventy-plus hours a week to achieve the lifestyle I was *taught* by the popular culture a private practice obstetrician was *supposed* to have. I had the Porsche, the big house, swimming pool, and a beautiful spouse. It didn't hurt that she was a physician in a lucrative practice also. I was living the American Dream. In fact, I was the American Dream.

One afternoon, and I remember this as clearly as I remember dinner yesterday evening, I was sitting by the swimming pool. The Midwestern sun was high in the clear, powder blue sky. A few billowy clouds were drifting listlessly on the horizon. "This is it," I said to myself. "This is it, I have arrived. I've reached the life I wanted, the light at the end of the tunnel, the life I struggled and trained for all of those years. I have it."

The emptiness in my belly was so profound that it consumed me. It rippled through me and swallowed my whole essence. I felt like a shell lying on a sandy beach, bright and shiny on the outside, completely empty, hollow, and lifeless on the inside. "This is to be the way I am going to live the rest of my life?" I asked myself. "This is it, and nothing more?"

There is more, so much more, but I did not understand that at the time. I did not understand what it meant to *need* to experience the Glow of Being Alive until I had arrived at what I thought was the end of the journey. The journey is all around us, and it is never ending. There is no beginning. There is no end. There is only an eternity of beauty, love, and experience open and available to each and every one of us–all we need to do is take it. We only need to embrace life, the experience of being alive, to the fullest, and the world, the universe, so to speak, is our oyster.

My personal journey to knowledge, or enlightenment, or whatever you want to call it, led me to the indigenous medicine traditions. These traditions of native cultures, the beauty ways of the peoples of the earth, are my personal spoke on the wheel in which truth with a capital "T" is at the center. This is a concept we will explore in the first chapter. The single, most important facet of life for indigenous peoples is to be in balance and harmony with themselves, with nature, and with our world. Without balance we succumb to dis-ease and illness. Without balance we wither away, struggling to *be* in ways that are not appropriate for us. It is *only* out of a place of balance and harmony that we arrive at our true nature, our true purpose, and are able to taste aliveness. It's only when we're in balance that we're able to achieve self-actualization and allow the beauty and majesty of the exquisite world we live in for so short a time to percolate through us. When we are in balance synchronicity and serendipity become operating principles in our lives. Struggle evaporates. Effort becomes an act of love and power. We live in vibrancy and walk within the Glow of Being Alive.

The Steps to Vibrancy are one method for wading through and stepping past the imprinting and conditioning our culture has heaped on us and arriving at our true nature, our true selves. They are six simple steps for reaching a state of self-actualization and arriving at the balance and harmony for which we are all searching. Simple, however, does not necessarily mean easy. Looking within ourselves and releasing those parts of ourselves that no longer serve us, that have been with us for as long as we can remember, is never easy. We share many memories and feelings with the attitudes, prejudices, and beliefs that we need to release. We have had many dinners with them, and saying good-bye to old friends is never easy. Yet sometimes we have to as we proceed along our own path, the path of beauty and fulfillment that is waiting for us as an individual. We each have one, one as unique as we are.

Engaging The Steps to Vibrancy will usher into motion processes which will forever alter the way you view yourself, the whole of creation, and the dynamics of your interactions with all of your relations--everyone and everything you share your life and world with. All of The Steps to Vibrancy and exercises should be engaged in as a ritual and in a ceremonial manner. The Steps to Vibrancy and exercises are *experiences* that access the divine, within and without, and the divine, the whole of creation, should always be treated as sacred. Don't just walk The Steps and do the exercises like schoolwork. Gift them to yourself as a precious act of love and power. Gift them to yourself, because you deserve whatever you desire.

The Circles of Emergence, the Fifth Step to Vibrancy, are a succinct paradigm for ordering our realities. They teach us that we truly do have the ability to choose, to choose anything we desire.

And that ability is terrifying when it becomes real. One of my mentors often says that it's one thing to talk about the ability to make it rain. It sounds good, and we think we would feel great if we could do it. It's quite another to do ceremony and then feel the cool rain cascading down over your face. Really owning the ability is terrifying, and the first time you make it rain, you'll probably pee in your pants.

Walking The Steps to Vibrancy will make you laugh, and will cause you to cry. They will kindle fears you never imagined, and teach you talents and gift you powers you never would have believed you possessed. The Steps to Vibrancy will take you beyond what you have been given by your upbringing, culture, and society. They will guide you past the concepts of duality, right and wrong, and past who and what you have been taught you are. Rumi, the Thirteenth Century Sufi poet, very succinctly tells us, "Out beyond our ideas of right doing, and wrong doing, there is a field. I'll meet you there." The Steps to Vibrancy guide us to that field. They will take you to the special place where there resides a majestic, radiant being who is you, and who is aglow with the same power of creation and divine beauty that informs galaxies and roses.

As we've said, each exercise in Living the Steps to Vibrancy is an experience. Each is a ritual and should be engaged in a ceremonial fashion. Ceremony and ritual have a way of focusing our intent and consciousness in a way that is beyond words. Through ceremony and ritual you tap into the energy and intent contained within the collective unconscious of those who have used the same processes for millennia to answer the same questions you are asking. When you engage the exercises in this fashion you are engaging archetypal processes which will become active in your life, and remain active long after you have completed that particular exercise.

Ceremony and ritual take us directly to the energetic level, and that's the place we need to reach for true and lasting change to occur.

Don't just sit down with a pad and paper when you come home from work and you're tired, or just whip out a pen as you're reading about the exercise and start writing in the margins of the book. Read what you are going to do. Understand what the exercise is about. Get a *feeling* for what the experience is attempting to do for you. Then set aside a quiet time. Take a bath. Go for a walk. Light candles. Make certain you won't be disturbed. Make it special. Make it sacred. Make it an act of love and an act of power. Then, and only then, begin, and engage the process with the intent to learn and see exactly what you need to learn and see.

There are as many paths to knowledge and enlightenment as there are spiritual disciples, and each of those paths is as valid as any other. Each contains the truth, the truth with a little "t." And each is an avenue to the center, the Truth with a capital "T." If a path works for you, use it. But don't become attached to it, because you will *experience*, as your consciousness expands and your view broadens, that all paths lead to the same place, the Source of All That Is. The Steps to Vibrancy are one path, and they are a framework in which to place your life in order to experience being alive, bring meaning to your life, and live in wholeness and Vibrancy–The Glow of Being Alive.

Unity

&

Separateness

Beyond that world of opposites is an unseen, but experienced unity and identity in us all.

Joseph Campbell

WE EXIST IN THE FIELD OF TIME AND SPACE, and a world of duality and separateness. This condition of duality and separateness is all that we know. Good–bad, up–down, sorrow–joy, here–there, is how our perception has been formed, and this perception is the only perception we know. Because we cannot remember experiencing anything except the world of opposites within the context of our conscious, linear lives, we think this is the only way there is, and we believe this is how everything in the universe is, seen and unseen.

We have all been given many, many sets of glasses since birth, lenses through which we view the world. These glasses come in the form of familial, cultural, and societal customs, taboos, prejudices, and rights and wrongs. Because we all have different glasses—no two people share the same exact set—*we all, each and every one of us, see the world with a slightly different focus.* This is easy to demonstrate. Get a group of people together. Give everyone a pencil and a sheet of white paper. Then ask the group to draw the color red. That's right! Ask everyone to draw the color red with only a pencil and a white sheet. You will see that everyone experiences what we all agree on as red differently. This seems mundane when we focus on a primary color. It's less mundane when we focus on the color of someone's skin.

Additionally, with the lenses we've been handed, we tend to focus on differences between things. We categorize all of the attributes of things, then we readily proceed to list all of the ways in which the things being compared are different. Our minds tell us that this is this, and, that is that, because they are different in ways x, y, and z.

Our focus on differences is again mundane, when, for example, we look at two coffee cups. This one is red. That one is white. This one has a square handle. That one has a round handle. This one has a picture of a cat. That one has a picture of a dog. The focus on differences becomes problematic when we take it to the level of people, communities, and religions. On these broader, encompassing levels, when we focus on differences and separateness we set up walls and barriers of exclusiveness. We enclose ourselves in boxes where we, and only we, have the truth. We, and only the exclusive group with which we share similar lenses have the *only way*. We isolate ourselves and then spend our lives struggling to keep ourselves separate from ***the other***.

The consequences of our focus on duality and differences is painfully evident when we look back through the pages of our history as a species. How many wars have been fought and how many lives spent supporting the walls of the box of separateness we have created for ourselves out of our perception of duality? How many religious leaders have preached of universal love and compassion, yet qualified their message by stating the necessity to be on ***their*** path to salvation and part of ***their*** in-group? Any religion of exclusion claiming to have the *only* truth, the truth with a capital "T" is a false religion–period.

The challenge for us as individuals and as a people, perhaps more important now than at any other point in history, is to change the lenses of our glasses. We need to remove the thick, clouded, scratched pieces of glass that focus our attention on differences and replace them with shiny, vibrant, translucent, panoramic lenses that see beyond the world of duality. Lenses that see into a universe of similarities, oneness, radiance and beauty.

In this book we are going to remove our worn lenses which constrict and narrow our view of ourselves, our lives, and our worlds, and slip on a pair of glasses which will shift our perception. We are going to put on glasses that broaden our perceptions of ourselves and our worlds. These are lenses that will focus our awareness and perception on commonalties and on abilities we never dreamed we possessed.

We'll begin by looking at the threads weaving together the world's great spiritual traditions, then extend that vision to the cutting edge of contemporary particle physics where the universe is becoming stranger and more mysterious than any science fiction writer ever imagined, and an arena where hard science and mysticism are mingling. A place where the distinction between subject and object entirely melts away, and pure subjectivity completely creates the mysterious environment we call home. Then, the thread of non-duality firmly in hand, we will extend our range of perception to broaden our view of ourselves through embodying The Steps to Vibrancy.

The Steps to Vibrancy teach us how to get to the place of Living in Vibrancy by broadening our view of ourselves, our world, our universe, and the whole of creation. First, we will step outside of the world of duality into a place of oneness recognized beneath the cultural milieu of all of the world's spiritual traditions, and then step back into the world of duality to live the life we ought to be living, fully energized and empowered by the knowledge and experience of our true potential.

This past summer I was walking the two dogs I share my life with, Dexter and Dakota, in the forest preserve near our home. As we were driving to the parking area closest to the trail where we like to begin our hikes, I saw a group of people playing baseball. They were in one corner of an expansive, flowing, green, grassy field that was at least 15 or 20 acres. They had the whole area to explore and enjoy, yet they had created boundaries in their world. The extent of their universe was demarcated with orange pylons. Everything beyond the pylons was out of bounds–it was all taboo. They had erected walls and separated their space from the universe which held them. Yet the whole of creation was there, just beyond their self-imposed boundaries, available, waiting, actually begging them to step over the threshold and explore.

The challenge of The Steps to Vibrancy is to throw away the orange pylons we set up for ourselves. The challenge is to throw away all of the boundaries of difference and separateness we have created for ourselves to explore a world and a universe so marvelous, mysterious, and beautiful that only a poet's verse can come close to describing it in a language we can understand. Though we may not understand through the words directly, we can **know** through the feelings the words stir within the depths of our bellies. The challenge is to cast away the pylons, explore, and then like Prometheus returning with the gift of fire, return to the world of duality, with the knowledge that we are so much more than we have been led to believe.

By Living in Vibrancy–The Glow of Being Alive, we share the gift of our internal fire with those with whom we share our lives, and our glow kindles the same spark that is within each and every one of us. Throw away the orange pylons, and enter *The Steps to Vibrancy*.

Come to the orchard in the spring
There is light and wine, and sweethearts
in the pomegranate flowers.
If you do not come, these do not matter.
If you do come, these do not matter.

Rumi

The Garden, The Fall
&
Separation

The wind, one brilliant day, called to my soul with
an odor of jasmine.
"In return for the odor of my jasmine, I'd like all the
odor of your roses."
"I have no roses; all the flowers in my garden are
dead."
"Well then, I'll take the withered petals and the
yellow leaves and the waters of the fountain."
The wind left. And I wept. And I said to myself:
"What have you done with the garden
that was entrusted to you?"

Antonio Machado

The Garden. The Serpent. Paradise lost. These images have become entrenched within our cultural unconscious and ingrained in the individual mental frameworks we use to engage the world. This preemptive strike to our unconscious has occurred whether or not we were raised in a religious household. Allusions to Eden, and Adam and Eve are ubiquitous in our popular culture. They are found in everything from advertising to sitcoms. I recently had a discussion with a close friend about this very point. She insisted it was not that apparent in our culture as a whole, and that since she was not raised in a religious household, she was not affected. Well, the very next day we were out in a car and stopped at a traffic light. What drives across the road in front of us? A bus with an advertisement on its side panel. The advertisement consisted of a giant apple with a bite taken out and the names Adam and Eve. You don't have to be religious in our culture to be part of the popular mythology.

We in Westernized cultures are the only people in the whole world who have ever been kicked out of the garden. This bears repeating. We in the West are the only people who have ever been cast out. We are the only people in whom the notion of separateness from nature is infused from birth. In fact, we're told we've been separated from nature even before we were born. We're told that we're born with original sin–a sin we acquired before we ever had the opportunity to do anything bad. And even worse, we're told that we have to spend our lives atoning for it! Our mythology, our Christian mythology–and I refer not to the true teachings and identity of the Christ Consciousness, but rather to how men have interpreted accounts of the teachings of Christ with the intent of controlling people–is a cultural guidepost, and an organizing force in our lives. We'll see as we walk through The Steps to Vibrancy how *conscious* our unconscious really is and how these cultural forces play an enormous role in our lives, whether we consciously believe in them or not.

"Out," the famous line of Genesis, Chapter 3 begins, "for you have eaten from the fruit of the tree of knowledge of good and evil." (For the purposes of this discussion we will not concern ourselves with the fact that many scholars consider the whole of Genesis to be a mistranslation of the Quabala, a true accounting of the mystical, unspeakable truths organizing the universe. The translation is what we've been taught. Since we've been told it's true and it's been wired into the syntax of our consciousness, it's what orders the way we view the world.) We're then told in Chapter 3 of Genesis that because we have tasted the fruit of the tree of knowledge of good and evil that woman, "...in pain you shall bring forth children," and man, "Cursed is the ground for your sake; in toil you shall eat of it all the days of your life." The serpent didn't escape this punitive deity's wrath either. The poor, misunderstood serpent was told, "...you are cursed more than all cattle, and more than every beast of the field; on your belly you shall go, and you shall eat dust all the days of your life." What a strange way of relating to nature! Come on, snakes aren't good or bad, they're just snakes. It's no wonder we're afraid of snakes and most everything else–we're taught to be afraid. But it gets worse.

Prior to the fall, in Chapter 1 of Genesis, man was given dominion over nature. "Fill the earth and subdue it," Adam was told. "Have dominion over the fishes of the sea, the birds of the air, and over every living thing that moves on the earth." Again, what a peculiar way of relating to the world, and to nature, which holds us so tenderly and is so intimately a part of our very being. Dominion over nature implies something completely different than the ideal of being a caretaker of nature, a notion the indigenous carry within their hearts and one we will embrace fully later in this chapter, and as we walk The Steps to Vibrancy.

Webster's dictionary defines dominion as: "The power or right of governing and controlling; sovereign authority." This notion of having the power and the right, the god given right no less, to control, implies a hierarchical system, and with us having been given top billing, it makes us better than what we have dominion over. These "rights" then make it easy for us to justify and absolve ourselves of guilt and responsibility for the rape and slaughter we have brought upon the planet. (I want to be clear that this chapter is not intended as a discussion of the historical accuracy of the Bible. It is intended, rather, as a review of how the lenses of our perception have been shaped and polished by the beliefs of our culture, and the stories and myths upon which we base our lives and interactions.)

Joseph Campbell considered mythologies and religions to be, "...great poems, and when recognized as such, point infallibly through things and events to the ubiquity of a 'presence' or 'eternity' that is whole and entire in each." For him, "The material of myth is the material of our life, the material of our body, and the material of our environment, and a living, vital mythology deals with these in terms that are appropriate to the nature of knowledge of the time." And on the nature of *reality* he succinctly explains that, "Reality is those myths we haven't quite seen through yet." Our worlds, our perceptions are ordered by those myths we have inherited, and in many cases these myths, these old ways of structuring reality, are no longer appropriate. They lose their life and vitality as our consciousness as a people changes and expands, and our views of reality and the paradigms with which we order the world shift.

The creation myth of Genesis, when taken as myth, and integrated in the context of the preceding definitions, indeed points to the same infallible truths, the same concepts of interconnectedness and oneness inherent in, and underlying every one of the world's great spiritual traditions, including, we shall see, the New Testament. The story of Genesis, when viewed through broader lenses of perception tells a stirring tale of oneness. Each of us, all of nature and existence, arose out of the same singular creative Source, the same potential of being, the same love. All of nature, including each of us, is part of that Source, and by being part of that potential, we share equally in its divinity. Genesis Chapter 1 emphatically states, "So God created man in His own image; in the image of God He created him; male and female He created them." God created *man* in

His *own image*. Look past the gender references in the statement. Our language is inadequate when trying to express pure beingness apart from gender.

Just as you cannot separate Mozart from his music, you cannot separate the creation from the creator. If we are created in God's image, how can we be anything less than God? To believe we are less is to heap upon ourselves great injustice and disempowers us beyond belief! Yet we have been taught, for the whole of our lives that we are so much less. It's no wonder we have so much difficulty believing in ourselves.

It's only when *we* create God in *our* image, and believe in this image concretely as Western religions do, that we get into trouble. Our linear thinking, rational minds cannot comprehend what is beyond words–those things that we can know and intuit, but cannot describe. Because we can't understand what's not understandable, we tend to bring the transcendent into the mundane instead of going beyond the mundane and stretching ourselves into the divine. In trying to make the incomprehensible comprehensible it's natural for us to translate the divine into something we can understand, and there is nothing we understand more, so we believe, than ourselves. By creating God in our image we give her all of our traits and qualities: love, beauty, and goodness are necessarily accompanied by control, anger, and judgment. However, because all of these notions have sprung from the same source, they all contain the creative potential. They are all divine. It's when we place judgment on them that we become troubled.

The Book of Twenty-four Philosophers, a 12th century text originally in Greek, describes God as: "An intelligible sphere," intelligible meaning known or sensed, but not understood, "whose center is everywhere, and circumference is nowhere." Think about this statement. Meditate with it. Let it slowly filter through your consciousness and allow it to carry you to a place beyond words. This description makes no sense to our rational mind, but it has the ability to pull us to the Godhead. If we allow it, it will carry us to The Source–the source of creativity and potential, the wellspring of each and every one of us, and the origin of all we know.

Let's now remove ourselves from the notion of separateness and the anthropomorphic nature of God, and return, in small steps, home to the realm of oneness and cohesiveness of which we are all part. There is no door, no impenetrable gate guarded by cherubim brandishing swords of fire. There is only a threshold. Join me in stepping across it, back into the Garden.

East & West
Two Points of The Same Circle

The East

"This that people say, 'Worship this god! Worship that god!'–one god after another! All this is his creation indeed! And he himself is all the gods....He is entered in the universe even to our fingernail-tips, like a razor in a razor case, or fire in firewood. This those people see not, for as seen he is incomplete. When breathing, he becomes 'breath' by name; when speaking, 'voice'; when seeing, 'the

eye'; when hearing, 'the ear'; when thinking, 'mind': these are but the names of his acts....

One should worship with the thought that he is one's self, for therein all these become one. This self is the footprint of that All, for by it one knows the All–just as, verily, by following a footprint one finds cattle that have been lost....One should reverence the Self alone as dear–what he holds dear, verily, will not perish.

So whosoever worships another divinity than his self, thinking, 'He is one, I am another,' knows not. He is like a sacrificial animal for the gods...."

Brihadaranyaka Upanishad

The passage above is from one of the earliest *Upanishads*, dating from about the 8th century BC. The *Upanishads* are early Hindu esoteric and mystical writings which are part of the *Veda*, one of six orthodox systems of Hindu philosophy. The *Vedanta*, composed of two Sanskrit words (*Veda*–knowledge, and, *Anta*–end) are concerned with the knowledge of *Brahman*, the universal, divine, supreme being. As we have discussed, it's difficult when writing or speaking about a God, Supreme Being, or Divine Intelligence not to anthropomorphize–give it human characteristics so we can relate to it and understand it. Even just calling it a being conjures up notions that it is somewhat like ourselves. Any human characteristics I may imply in this book are purely the result of inadequacies in our language.

The *Upanishads* seek to explain the intimate relationship between *Brahman*, the universal intelligence, creative source, or spirit, with the individual self, breath, or soul–*Atman*. The concept of breath or air as the animating factor in all of life, or as the soul, is also inherent to notions of our ultimate nature held by native peoples.

According to the *Upanishads*, as interpreted by the Hindu philosopher Shankara, *Brahman* and *Atman* are identical. There is not only no separation, but there is **no difference** between the source of all creation, us, and everything around us. And everything means just that–*every thing*. We are part of everything, and part of the nature we walk in. And everything, including the magnificent natural world we live in, is part of us. We truly are *Children of the Earth*.

In other Hindu philosophies it's stated that until you understand that God is everything–*every thing*–and everywhere, you will remain cloaked in the veil of *Maya*. *Maya* in this context means illusion and ignorance. Everything means, simply, *every thing*. This cannot be over stated. You just cannot separate the creator from the creation–they are one and the same. They are one in the same whole. God, the creative source, is in, simply *is*, everything. God is every stone, every plant, every piece of metal, every drop of water, every mineral, and every one of us. God is also all that we would consider filth. Every piece of what we call garbage is creation, including every noxious odor, every rotting vegetable, any kind of trash we can imagine. It's all God. It's all creation! We tend to only associate God with what we like and deem as good. But that's merely a judgment we place on things because some things serve our egos and some do not. Judgment is a powerful attribute we've given ourselves that we will explore in depth in The Steps to Vibrancy. God is everything, and everything is God. One has to embrace it all!

An Eastern mystic was once asked, "Since all is *Brahman*, all is the divine radiance, how can we say 'no' to ignorance or brutality? How can we say 'no' to anything?" He answered his pupil: "For you and I, we say 'yes.'" We have to embrace everything, because *every thing* is creation. Everything is beauty. Everything is love. And this love is not the sentimental love we're used to, but something that goes far beyond our words and usual experience. This is the unconditional love of creator for creation. This love is the Source of All. It is the wellspring of everything, and the binding force that holds everything together.

This idea comes across crystal clear in the *Upanishads*, and we will see it present in all of our spiritual traditions. In the *Upanishads*, the individual soul, or breath, is identical to the universal breath, or spirit, but the individual soul does not understand its real or non-dual nature because of ignorance–*avidya*. And we see this exact theme presented in the Bible. John 1:4–5 can be translated as, "...the life is the light of man. And the light shines in darkness: and the darkness comprehends it not." The light, *Brahman*, the eternal, the divine, shines in us, the darkness. The darkness is us, our ego identity. We are veiled by *Maya*, illusion, to our true nature. And the darkness, us, comprehends it not. We do not comprehend the divinity within ourselves.

Ignorance, or the power of illusion, *Maya*, inherent in and projected from *Brahman* is what masks the universality of *Brahman* and causes us to only experience things as separate from ourselves. It's what makes us define our world in terms of ourselves and *the other*, everything other than ourselves. It's because of our perception of ourselves as separate from *the other* that we experience the world of suffering–*Samsara*. In Hindu philosophy it's taught that through proper study of the *Veda* we can realize our true, limitless nature and the cohesive, non-dual, non-separate nature of the ultimate reality. It's through this sacred union we understand that we are identical to *Brahman* and reach a state of *nirvana*, or bliss.

This concept of all pervading unity, oneness, and sameness with The Source is also seen in the Hindu holy text *The Bhagavad*

Gita, which is translated as, *The Song of The Lord*. *The Bhagavad Gita* is a Sanskrit poem set in Book VI of the epic *Mahabharata*. It is a dialogue between the incarnate god *Krishna* and *Prince Arjuna*. In the poem they discuss the nature of the soul and the proper way to reach God.

In *The Bhagavad Gita, Krishna* states:

> *"Such as one grows to oneness with Brahman;*
> *Such as one growing on with Brahman, serene,*
> *Sorrows no more, desires no more; his soul,*
> *Equally loving all that lives, loves well*
> *Me, Who have made them, and attains to Me....*
> *How, if thou hearest that the man new–dead*
> *Is, like the man new-born, still living man–*
> *One same, existent Spirit–wilt thou weep?*
> *The end of birth is death; the end of death*
> *Is birth: this is ordained!"*

Krishna continues:

> *"He that had meditated on Me alone*
> *In putting off his flesh, comes forth to Me,*
> *Enters into my being–doubt that not!...*
> *Who, offering sacrifice of wakened hearts,*
> *Have sense on one pervading Spirit's stress,*
> *One force in every place, though manifold...*
> *I am–of all of this boundless universe–*
> *The Father, Mother, Ancestor, and Guard...."*

And *Krishna* concludes:

> *"Death am I, and immortal Life am I,*
> *Arjuna! Visible Life,*
> *And Life invisible."*

Indeed, *every thing* is creation. Each of us is creation. And each of us is creator!

Buddhism, based largely on the Hindu tradition, retains and embodies the concept of the oneness of all creation. Buddhist doctrine clearly describes that we all, and in fact everything surrounding us not only contains, but *is the creative potential*. While most of Buddhist doctrine is concerned with the illusory nature of the material world, and a path to overcoming our ignorance of the true nature of reality by stepping past our ego identity into nirvana, the concept of Dependent Origination brings forth the idea of oneness of all creation.

In the Buddhist system, the whole universe, all of creation, has simply arisen. All that is has simply come into existence from one Source, or potential. The symbol for this is the lotus blossom which has arisen out of an infinitely deep pond and floats quiescent upon the surface of the pond's still water. The petals are not to be interpreted singularly, but as parts of the same whole. And that whole is a reflection of The Source beneath the water on which the blossom floats. The Dependent Origination of Consciousness essentially states that our consciousness arises out of our interaction with the world of forms, corporeality, and that this consciousness is transient.

An early Buddhist text, *The Word of Buddha*, indicates the Buddha explained, "...the arising of consciousness is dependent upon conditions; and without these conditions, no consciousness arises." And, "It is impossible that any one can explain the passing out of one existence, and entering into a new existence, ...independent of corporeality, feeling, perception, and mental formations." The Buddha then further states, "All formations are 'transient'...," even, "Corporeality is transient...."

In essence, the Dependent Origination of Consciousness simply states that we exist because of our relationships. There is no independent existence. Without something to be related to there can be no being. Beingness, including our own existence, is dependent on there being other beings and things to be related to. Think about it. If nothing else existed, how could you be? We are defined by our relationships to other things, and we will explore this in depth while walking The Steps to Vibrancy.

What this all points to is the singular Source from which all of creation arises, the interconnectedness of all things at the most basic, elemental level, and the subjective nature of reality. In essence, *we create reality*, something we'll see is now being proven by modern physics.

For Buddhist philosophy the idea of *Anatman* is central, and is related to Dependent Origination. The doctrine of *Anatman* teaches that there is no permanent soul. Our idea of a permanent soul is illusory and arises out of Dependent Origination, our ego creating the world around us, and its desire not to die. Once the idea of a permanent soul is transcended, we realize that all things are without a self. All things are a manifestation of transcendence. All things are Buddha things. This is not to say that there is not a you or a me. It's just that you and I are more than we can ever imagine. There is a you and I, but just like waves are part of the ocean, we are part of something larger and more encompassing than we can comprehend. The you and the I are *every thing!*

The Buddha states: "There is, oh monks, a state where there is neither earth, nor water, nor air; neither infinity of space nor infinity of consciousness, nor nothingness, nor perception nor non-perception; neither this world nor that world, neither sun nor moon. ...it is the eternal which never originates and never passes away."

The idea of reaching *nirvana*, the place of transcendence "...which never originates and never passes away," and yet maintaining an ego identity is one of the ideas encompassed in the ideal of the Bhodisattava–an enlightened being who forgoes melting back into the great pool of consciousness and returns to the world to aid others in the path to enlightenment. Later in this chapter we will see a similar concept echoed in the indigenous medicine teachings where a medicine person strives to activate their luminous body and differentiate into a luminous being–a being who maintains identity yet transcends the world of duality and the field of time and space.

Echoes of our oneness with, and the unity of all creation are seen in writings and traditions as diverse as *The Analects of Confucius*, *The Egyptian Book of The Dead*, and within the Greco-Roman tradition.

The Analects of Confucius, though primarily concerned with social order in society, reflect an underlying spiritual theme. Speaking to one of his disciples, Confucius says, "Shan, my doctrine is that of an all-pervading unity." Confucius leaves, and Tsang, another disciple, clarifies his words to the other students. Tsang explains, "The doctrine of our master is to be true to the principles of our nature and the benevolent exercise of them to others, this and nothing more." We are to realize, and live out of, a sense of oneness and all-pervading unity. This is a theme sorely needed in *our* politics and social structuring.

In *The Egyptian Book of The Dead* it's stated: "I, even I, am a Spirit-soul, a dweller in the Light-god, whose form hath been created in divine flesh." It goes on to say, "My moment is in your bodies, but my forms are in my place of habitation. I am 'He who cannot be known.'" The theme of a unity and oneness with Source is again clearly apparent, as is the idea that we are not to be seen as separate from the Source, but that we, in fact, *are* The Source, and that The Source can be realized, but not known to our intellect.

The Egyptian Book of The Dead also contains a long passage regarding transmigration and changing forms. This passage, too lengthy to reproduce here, again points to the universality of all things by virtue of all things being able to transform into all other things.

In *Metamorphosis*, Ovid, the Roman poet (43BC–AD17?) relates the teachings of the Sage, Samos. *Metamorphosis* is an epic poem which charts the history of the world from creation to the time of Julius Caesar, and emphasizes the inherent instability and changing nature of the world. Samos, Ovid writes, taught, "All things change, but they are one. The one wax takes many molds."

The West

All of us living beings belong together in as much as we are all in reality sides or aspects of one single being, which may perhaps in western terminology be called God while in the Upanishads its name is Brahman.

Physicist Erwin Schrodinger

Western thought and religion has been structured almost entirely by what we call the Judeo-Christian tradition, yet to refer to what has become the overriding mythic structure of the Western world as "Judeo-Christian" is somewhat of a misnomer. As noted ecologist and philosopher, David Abram, points out in his acclaimed book, *The Spell of The Sensuous*:

> "We moderns tend to view ancient Hebraic culture through the intervening lens of Greek and Christian thought; even Jewish scholarship, and much contemporary Jewish self-understanding, has been subtly influenced and informed by centuries of Hellenic and Christian interpretation. It is only thus that many persons today associate the ancient Hebrews with such anachronistic notions as the belief in an otherworldly heaven and hell, or a faith in the immateriality and immortality of the personal soul. Yet such dualistic notions have no real place in the Hebrew bible. Careful attention to the evidence suggests that the ancient Hebraic religiosity was far more corporeal, and far more responsive to the sensuous earth, than we commonly assume."

Mr. Abram proceeds to points out that in the Hebrew Bible, the word *ruach*, which in Hebrew means both spirit and wind, is the omnipresent force of creation which gives rise to everything, and is *in everything*. In the Hebrew Bible, known as the *Tanakh: The Holy Scriptures*, Genesis 1:2 can be translated as, "When God began to create heaven and earth–the earth being unformed and void, with darkness over the surface of the deep and a wind–*ruach*–from God sweeping over the water...."

The intent here is only to suggest that the roots of contemporary Judaism are much more animate, nature centered, and soulful than we have commonly been led to believe. It is also critical to note that in the Judeo-Christian tradition, as is seen in all cultures, the God commonly described and worshipped is an anthropomorphization–a God created in the images of men–and its form is intimately related to the cultural milieu in which it was conceived.

The New Testament and the teachings of Christ also fall prey to our inherent tendency to create God in our image and view words and deeds through the perception of the culture at large. The words, teachings, and parables of Christ, when viewed through broader lenses describe the same oneness, the same divinity, and the same creative source within all of creation, including within each one of us, as we see in the Eastern traditions and indigenous cultures.

The Gnostic Gospels, known as the *Nag Hammadi Library*, named after the area in upper Egypt where they were discovered in 1945, are a group of religious texts written in the first few centuries after the death of Jesus. They constitute a broader, more affirming, empowering, and mystical interpretation of the teachings of Christ than given in the traditional, sanctified, sanitized bible of the Christian Church. Since the Gnostic Gospels don't fit with the main stream, bureaucratic, and controlling thinking of the present day Christian Church, they are considered heretical, and viewed with askance.

In the Gnostic Gospel according to the disciple Thomas, Jesus said, "Whoever drinks from my mouth shall become as I am and I myself will become he, and the hidden things shall be revealed to him... I am the All, the All came forth from me and the All attained to me. Cleave a piece of wood, I am there; lift up the stone and you will find me there." This is the exact sentiment, the same heartfelt thought, reflected in the passage from the Upanishads we read earlier! God is everything. Everything is God. All, including God, is an act of divine creation, and all, *all of creation*, holds the singular, creative potential within itself.

31

The theme of oneness is further expounded upon by Jesus. Jesus is reported by Thomas to have said:

"Rather, The Kingdom [of God] is inside of you, and it is outside of you. When you come to know yourselves, then you will become known, and you will realize that it is you who are the sons of the living father....When you make the two one, and when you make the inside like the outside and the outside like the inside, and the above like the below, and when you make the male and the female one and the same, so that the male not be male nor the female female...then will you enter [the kingdom]....It [the kingdom] will not come by waiting for it. It will not be a matter of saying 'here it is' or 'there it is.' Rather, the kingdom of the father is spread upon the earth, and men do not see it."

Didn't we see this same thought a few pages ago as written by John? "And the light shines in darkness: and the darkness comprehends it not."

It can't be any clearer. The knowledge, the creative potential, The Source is within each of us, within everything, within every being. And The Source, the Godhead transcends the world of duality, the field of time and space. The kingdom is here. We're in it. This is it! This *is* the kingdom. This *is* the garden. We, however, are blinded by ignorance and conditioning and don't recognize that we're not only surrounded by divinity, but we *are* divinity.

Examining the traditional Bible with our new lenses of perception we also find this same theme. In the Epistle of Paul to the Colossians 3:10–11, we find: "And have put on the new man who is renewed in knowledge according to the image of Him who created him, Where there is neither Greek nor Jew...but Christ is all and in all." Christ is all, and in all. And, all is in Christ. All of creation is imbued with the Christ Light. All things are Buddha things. We are, every one of us, not only part of the Christ light, but, in truth, **are** the Christ Light. We are one with the Christ Light because we are the Christ Light; we just don't realize it. This notion, though alien to us, is taken for granted in Oriental cultures where we are all considered to be Gods waiting to achieve self-realization.

It should be more than crystal clear, but in our subjugation and degradation of ourselves, and by separating and alienating ourselves from nature, a natural world that we are intimately a part of, we've missed it. The Kingdom of God, the Creative Source, the realm of potential and being is not somewhere else. Eternity is not somewhere else. The infinite is not somewhere else. The kingdom is right here, all around us in this beautiful, interactive, sensual world. We only have to open our eyes and our hearts to experience the kingdom. All we need to do is change our perception. Perception is everything. We only need to change the tired, worn glasses through which we have learned to view the world in order to experience the divinity surrounding us, and within us.

We're living in *the kingdom* right now! This message is prevalent throughout the traditional Bible, we just have to open our eyes and shed light upon the darkness to see it. And the message of the Bible, when pried apart from the cultural milieu in which it was conceived, is one of beauty, love, and oneness with Source. The Apostle John, Chapter 14:10-11, writes of Jesus speaking about the unknowable oneness. "Do you not believe that I am in the Father, and the Father in Me? The words that I speak to you I do not speak on My own *authority*; but the Father who dwells in Me does the works. Believe Me that I am in the Father and the Father in Me, or else believe Me for the sake of the works themselves." And in 14:20 John writes that Jesus said, "...you will know that I am in My Father, and you in Me, and I in you."

It really can't be any clearer. All of our great, time honored, Eastern and Western mystical and spiritual traditions tell us the same thing. Their languages are different, and the images of their myths and metaphors vary, but underneath it all, their voices are the same. They all share in delivering to us the same message of beauty and oneness, and of divinity within, and without. They all inform us that we are in God, the Divine Source and creative potential, and this Source is in us—**in each of us!**

The Indigenous Tribal Wisdom Long Forgotten

As we are part of the land, you too are part of the land. The earth is precious to us. It is also precious to you. One thing we know: There is only one God. No man, be he Red Man or White Man can be apart. We are brothers after all.

Chief Seattle

The indigenous haven't forgotten. The indigenous haven't been kicked out of the garden. They live in it. They care for it. They are a part of it, and it's a part of them. Chief Seattle (Seathl), in his speech of 1855, when he was forced to give up his tribal lands said, "Man did not weave the web of life, he is merely a strand in it. Whatever he does to the web, he does to himself."

The native peoples around the world know. They know that we are not separate from anything. They know we are part of *every thing*. They know we are one small part of a whole more magnificent and grand than we can imagine. But we have lost touch with our Source. We have lost touch with ourselves. We have distanced ourselves and separated ourselves from the nature and divinity around us.

Try this experience. Go outside on a clear night and look up into the sky. You should preferably not be near a large city where a lot of light pollution will cloud your view. Gaze up into the dark sky and allow yourself, your inner self, to expand and be free. What do you feel? What do you see? You see a vastness which extends beyond any imagination you can have, and more stars than the greatest of our super computers can count. I was doing this one night, gazing up into an inky black sky speckled with tiny pinpoints of blue-white light, and I was reminded of a line from one of the Star Trek movies. It was the final scene of the film and Captain Kirk is asked what heading he wants. Where does he want to go? He waves his hand casually and says, "Out there, somewhere." See, the thing is, we **are** out there somewhere. There is not an **out there** and a **here** where we are the center of the universe–even though we still tend to think that's the case.

The thought that we are the center of the universe should have been banished from our consciousness when we finally admitted that the earth revolves around the sun. Unfortunately we really haven't accepted this. We still perceive ourselves as the center of the universe and believe everything is beholden to us. We are, in truth, not the center of anything. We really are *out there somewhere*. We are out there floating within a vastness we can't imagine. Our sun is out there too, one of zillions of stars, inhabiting zillions of galaxies. And our own universe is perhaps one of an infinitude of universes. We've forgotten that we are out there. The indigenous have not.

Indigenous cultures across the globe universally recognize that we are *out there*, and that we, as Chief Seattle so eloquently states, "...are merely a strand in the web of life." We are but one part of a large picture, and our actions affect the whole ball of wax. What happens when we don't recognize this? "What will happen when the buffalo are all slaughtered?" Chief Seattle continues. "The wild horses tamed? ...Where will the eagle be? Gone! ...The end of living and the beginning of survival." A dear friend reviewing the manuscript of this work commented on this paragraph. In the margin she wrote, "We are there."

Tribal peoples universally recognize the earth as a sentient, conscious, feeling being. For native peoples the earth is our mother. She is our true mother. She is conscious, aware, and responsive to us. She, like us, feels pain. She experiences hardships and suffers. Native peoples treat our Mother Earth with the respect we're taught to have for our biologic mother.

And in a very real, physical sense, the earth is our mother. Our physical bodies, though processed through our biologic mother, came from the earth. Everything that makes up our physical body is of the earth. All of the food we eat which becomes our physical body originates from the earth. In fact, everything that we encounter in our daily lives, from the book you're reading, to your car, your pager and your computer, to the stove in your kitchen and the sink in your bathroom, everything we use has come from the earth. Talk about oneness! Everything is made of the same stuff! We don't recognize it as such because we've distanced ourselves from the collection and processing of the raw materials. But everything comes from the earth, the Mother Earth.

In the Andean medicine traditions the earth is called the *Pachamama* and she is treated with respect and adoration. She is the being that provides for us, and holds us, and without whom we would not survive. As Carol Cumes points out in her book, *Pachamama's Children*, the natives of Peru "see Her (Pachamama) outside of themselves and inside of themselves as well. They see Her everywhere, in the wind that carries the clouds, in the clouds that bring the needed rains and in the sacred rivers that flow through the land. They see Her in the faces of their children and in the eyes of the puma, the condor, and the serpent." They also understand very clearly that, "If there is no *Pachamama* there cannot be a humanity nor a plant or animal kingdom."

In native North American traditions the earth is also adored, respected, and considered our true mother. She is conscious and a part of us. And we are part of her. When one enters a *Kiva*, an underground chamber used by the Hopi for sacred ceremonies, one is considered to be returning to the womb. The same is true of the sweat lodge ceremony, not unique to native North Americans, but common to native traditions around the world. Entering the lodge is considered a returning to the womb of the mother where you are purified and then *reborn* into the world.

This theme is woven through all of the North American indigenous traditions: Hopi, Navaho, Zuni, Sioux, etc. There is a Zuni story of emergence which says that when we came upon this earth, it was just like a child being born from its mother. And when we pass on, we return to our mother. "I am," a Pawnee man who has died and now returns as a ghost begins, "in everything; in the grass, the water." All native cultures recognize our oneness with the earth and all things.

Look at any indigenous culture from anywhere in the world and you will see the earth, the Mother Earth, treated with the respect and adoration of a sentient being who takes care of her children. We are part of the earth, we are her offspring, and we are intimately related to her. We were not dropped here from above, but have been birthed from her womb. We physically are *children of the earth*, and with this knowledge we can understand why the ways of the indigenous have been called, "The beauty ways of the peoples of the earth."

One of the most beautiful and stirring passages I have ever read about adoration of the Mother Earth come from Carlos Casteneda, in his wonderful book *Tales of Power*. Castenada and another shaman apprentice are in the desert with the shaman-sorcerers Don Juan and Don Genaro. It's nighttime and Castenada is complaining that the path they're on–the path of a sorcerer–is very lonely. Don Juan tells him to look at Genaro. Castenada turns and sees a ball of light swimming within a much larger ball of luminosity. Don Juan tells Castenada:

> "Only if one loves this earth with unbending passion can one release one's sadness. A warrior is always joyful because his love is unalterable and his beloved, the earth, embraces him and bestows upon him inconceivable gifts. The sadness belongs only to those who hate the very thing that gives shelter to their beings. This lovely being, which is alive to its last recesses and understands every feeling, soothed me, it cured me of my pains, and finally when I had fully understood my love for it, it taught me freedom."

It's only once we learn respect for the being who takes care of us, down to every last detail, that we will realize this is it–*this is the garden*. We're not only in it, we are part of it. And being a caretaker of something or someone is entirely different than having dominion over something or someone. We need to learn to be caretakers of the *Pachamama*, the marvelous being who takes care of us; for, as Carol Cumes points out, "If there is no *Pachamama* there cannot be a humanity nor a plant or animal kingdom."

The concept of oneness is inherent to every indigenous culture. Since we are all *of the Pachamama*, we're all part of the same source, and we're all made of the same stuff. It is purely our ideas of duality and separation that keep us trapped within the miserable self-image we've given ourselves. John Perkins, former CEO of a major US energy company, and a frequent consultant to the World Bank, United Nations, and Fortune 500 companies, has worked with the shamans of Ecuador for over thirty years. For him, and for them, many of our problems are wrapped up in our concept of *the other*.

For us, and our ego identity, there is a *me*, and there is everything else, *the other*. The renowned Swiss psychologist, Carl Jung, approximated this idea with his concept of the shadow. Our shadow, in very simplistic terms, is everything that we are not, or don't consider ourselves to be capable of being. Our shadow is all of the things we aren't, good or bad. The indigenous take this concept one step further, into the world of spirit, consciousness, and energy. For the shamans of Ecuador, as well as shamans around the globe, there is no *other*. There just *is*. Everything is one, and everything is energy. The reason we have trouble accepting this is because we are so attached to who we are. In his book *Shapeshifting*, John Perkins is having a discussion about shapeshifting and *the other* with a South American shaman. The shaman tells Mr. Perkins, "You know very well how they do it [shapeshift]. They don't really become this other at all, because all along they were this other. They and it are the same." Once we relinquish the concept of *the other*, we can step into whoever or whatever we desire to be because we are not separate or different from anything.

The shaman then proceeds to clarify his point. "Energy. It is everything. We are energy. The earth, those trees down there, this pyramid. The universe. Energy. That is all there is to it. It's just that ancient people were much closer to their physical world." Everything is made of the same stuff, and this stuff has been called many things. It has been called Buddha stuff, and the Christ Light. Now, many people call it Energy.

The idea that everything is energy is not merely a New Age conceptualization. Seers and medicine people have been telling us that everything is energy for millennia. Seers describe the universe as composed of fibers of light connecting everything to every other thing. They say that not only is everything connected by these fibers of light, but that everything, including us, is composed of these fibers of light. This is not simply a conceptualization, this is a reality. It's a reality which can be engaged just the same as when we write a letter or pick up the phone.

On a recent journey to Peru a woman was gifted a stone by one of the medicine people who had performed ceremonies for the group she was traveling with. The highland medicine people in Peru live high in the Andes, and the *Apus*–the mountains and the spirits of the mountains–are sacred to them. Stones are also sacred to the medicine people and considered power objects–objects that form a link to the strength and wisdom of the mountains. For some reason the stone gifted to the woman fell out of her back pack. She didn't realize that the stone had fallen out of her bag until she had returned from the day trip and was back at base camp and in her tent. The woman searched without success. She didn't hold any hope of ever recovering the lost gift.

The next day a medicine woman arrived at the traveler's tent. This medicine woman was not the same person with whom she had done the ceremonies, nor was this woman even around when she was given the stone the day before. The medicine woman rattled the tent. When the traveler stepped out, the medicine woman handed her the stone that had fallen out of her backpack the day before. The woman was stunned. She was shocked. She asked the medicine woman how she knew stone belonged to her? How had she found her? The medicine woman casually replied that she found the stone lying on the ground and merely followed the thread of light back to the woman's tent.

Quantum Physics
Closing the Circle

...we are to recognize in this whole universe a reflection magnified of our own most inward nature; so that we are indeed its ears, its eyes, its thinking, and its speech–or, in theological terms, God's ears, God's eyes, God's thinking, and God's word; and, by the same token, participants here and now in an act of creation that is continuous in the whole infinitude of that space of our mind through which the planets fly, and our fellows of earth now among them.

Joseph Campbell

Some Peruvian Shamans use the metaphor of closing a circle. The say that we lose energy and drain ourselves because we open circles–relationships, thoughts, ideas, activities, emotions–and never close them. We never bring closure to what we've begun. This is one of the reasons we become ill and at dis-ease. We don't close issues thereby leaving ourselves in an unbalanced state. Modern quantum physics is in many ways closing the circles we left open when we gave up an animate, spirit-filled world view for a mechanistic paradigm. Newton and his laws of motion had a tremendous effect on our perception by cementing into our consciousness the mechanistic view of the world and universe which began with Descartes and the Cartesian model of reality. However, with Einstein's arrival and his General and Special theories of relativity, the set, defined, and orderly world of subject and object was spun around, and a return to a more animate universe had begun. Quantum physics is now in many ways reanimating the world and returning spirit to us.

For me it is especially fulfilling and a real closure. When I was younger I wanted desperately to be a physicist, but I did not enjoy the math. The dry formulas and equations bored me to tears. I wanted to be a physicist because I believed that through physics I could answer the four big questions presented in the introduction of this book. Through the formulas and computations, I thought I could answer the real questions of the soul. Today, I am somewhat of a mystic, and I am in awe at how physics and mysticism are mingling and arriving at the same truths with a capital "T" from different spokes on the same wheel. In fact, today there is little difference between the postulates of theoretical physics and what mystics have been telling us for millennia.

A complete description of modern quantum physics is beyond the scope of this book, and indeed not necessary. I am only going to point out a couple of the ways in which our *hard* science is softening, entering the domains of heart and soul, and bringing us back to the spiritual nature that is our essence.

All of the spiritual traditions recognize many different kinds of time. We, within the context of our physical lives, have only experienced one type of time–linear time that flows like an arrow. Now you might say it's absurd to think of any other kind of time. Time is time–that's it. How can there be anything else? We think this way because linear time is the only time we have ever experienced, and it's the only kind of time our linear minds can comprehend. In the spiritual traditions there is another kind of time–and again, this is universal to all spiritual traditions whether they are indigenous or mystical.

This different kind of time has many names, and has been described in many different ways. It's been called sacred time, polychronic time, the eternal now, no-time. It is envisioned as time that folds back on itself, or time that is circular. In this alternate time everything that has, can, and will ever happen is present in an eternal moment of now. This statement doesn't seem to make sense, is difficult for us to comprehend, and impossible for us to intellectualize. But this kind of time is real, I assure you, and you will experience it when you reach the fourth Step to Vibrancy and Step Into the Empty Space.

What is fascinating is that modern physics is now postulating this kind of circular time. Stephen Hawking is considered by most physicists to be the most brilliant man since Einstein. Hawking, who brought to popular consciousness the concept of black holes, and though, from most perceptions, is crippled with a debilitating neurological disease, continues to bring forth the most provocative theories of our era. In one of his latest theories regarding the origin of the universe, he postulates what he calls imaginary time. He describes imaginary time as time that is not linear as we are used to, but instead circular. He describes it as time that folds back on itself. And he has the math to make it work! With our modern tools he has arrived at the same place mystics have been leading those who dared to go for centuries.

Mystics and seers have also been giving us physical descriptions of the universe–the energetic universe they *see*. For millennia seers have been describing the universe they *see* as composed of luminous filaments of light. They *see* the universe as fibers of conscious light, in a majestic, unimaginable tapestry connecting everything to everything. Everything is not only connected by these fibers of light, the fibers of light are the actual substance, the stuff that is the essence of everything.

The shamans of Peru consider themselves weavers. When they do their work, they say that they are weaving together the threads of light that interconnect everything. In the cloths they weave, they weave in universal energy patterns that they *see*. In fact, tools they use in their shamanic work resemble knitting needles. They use them for teasing and weaving the filaments of light binding all of creation together.

Physics is not only concerned with the origin of the universe, but with how everything works–how it all fits together. Physicists have a new theory about how things are. They call it the theory whose time hasn't come because it is so complex that even with our super computers there is no one alive today who can comprehend the math. The theory is known as the Super String Theory. This theory postulates that the universe is composed of infinitesimally tiny strings of conscious, vibrating light. These strings are so tiny that if an atom were expanded to the size of the known universe, it would be composed of zillions of these strings, and they would still be infinitesimally small. These strings not only connect everything to every other thing, they are what everything is made of. One thing can't be affected without affecting the whole because everything is linked together and made of the same stuff. Another circle closed.

Physics has even reached into the realm of oneness the spiritual traditions speak about where the relationship between subject and object disappear. As we have seen, all is one, and the world we're used to is merely a projection, something we create. Remember the concept of *Maya*. There is no definite subject–object relationship, there is only subject–subject. There can be no pure subject and pure observer, because the act of observing changes the subject. In other words, the act of observing creates what we are seeing. This is a critical concept that we will understand fully and embody within The Steps to Vibrancy. Physics has shown this, and actually proven it to be true. This truth is contained in what is known as the Heisenberg Uncertainty Principle. In simplistic terms, terms that avoid the math, the Uncertainty Principle holds that *the act of knowing affects that which is known*. We cannot know something without becoming part of what we are trying to know, and that becoming part of what we want to know affects it. For a thorough description of the physicist's approach to this whole concept I refer you to a wonderful book, *The Self-Aware Universe,* written by physicist Amit Goswami, Ph.D.

This first chapter has been the completion of a circle. We have in a sense closed a circle by traveling the globe in space and time, and *seeing* that the underlying themes of oneness, beauty, and creative potential held within each of us are present everywhere. The idea that the creative potential is present in everything, and is *every thing*, including us, is inherent to every single mystical tradition. This is clearly apparent when the archaic and anachronistic cultural and societal taboos and dogma which men have heaped onto traditions of beauty out of fear and the need for power and control over others are removed. We have also seen that we are now returning with the aid of our modern tools, to the place of the mystic, because this place cannot be avoided. Our modern myths of quantum particles are returning us to the realm of oneness and connection with everything because that's *what is at the center of the wheel*. It's our Source.

The real power, the power of beauty and creation and unlimited potential is within each and every one of us. Let's now walk The Steps to Vibrancy and realize how to bring that limitless potential and power into our lives, and re-empower ourselves by reconnecting with our Source.

The Steps to Vibrancy

Take Responsibility

Get Into Your Power

Eliminate Excuses

Step Into The Empty Space

Choose Your Circle

Vibrancy: The Glow of Being Alive

ONE

Take Responsibility

The world is a dream, dreamed by a single dreamer,
where all of the dream characters dream too.

Arthur Shopenhauer

THE GERMAN PHILOSOPHER SCHOPENHAUER is speaking about our world and universe. He is referring to the totality of what we consider reality, not only the dream worlds we visit in our sleep. In his intriguing statement where each of us is the single dreamer, he mimics knowledge native peoples have known forever. John Perkins, world business consultant turned shaman, in *The World Is As You Dream It: Shamanic Teachings from* *the Amazon and Andes*, describes how the indigenous of Ecuador believe that everything that occurs in our lives, every event that we participate in, happens first in our dreams. They believe we manifest our reality by dreaming it first. This belief is echoed in cultures as diverse as the Aborigine of Australia who describe The Dream Time, the place from which our world originated and continues to manifest, to the Eskimo of Siberia who speak about worlds, real worlds like ours, created by the *intent* of those who live in and visit them. Mystical traditions from across the globe all tell us there is a realm of intuition and wholeness where we act, live, love, experience, and even die and are reborn which is separate from the common, ordinary, and consensual reality we're used to.

These *dream peoples* also believe that we can focus and control our dreaming attention. Just as we've seen that there are different sorts of time, there are varying types of awareness and perception. The awareness or attention that we make use of in our dreams is different, but parallel to the awareness or attention we use in our everyday world. The attention and consciousness we have in our dream states is just as valid and real as the consciousness and awareness we use to perceive the everyday world. It is merely a different form of awareness.

By becoming aware of this dream consciousness, or attention, and learning to exercise volition with it, we can live in our dreams just the same as we do in our everyday lives. As dream explorers have so succulently explained, "There is nothing in the world that you can do to prove that you're not dreaming right now." This statement is very true. Think about it. Try proving to yourself that you're not dreaming right now. You can't! If you have ever had a very lucid dream then you know that the feelings, emotions, and actions in that dream state were just as sensual and real as those that occur in your everyday, waking life.

50

As we explore The Steps to Vibrancy we'll see that this dreaming attention is the same awareness that envelops us when we are meditating, traveling on a shamanic journey, or creating from within The Empty Space. This awareness is an ability we all have. It's a natural ability, but one that we've not been taught to foster. It's the same awareness that shamans use to *see*, and to meet and dialogue with their spirit guides. And it's the same awareness that we use to see angels.

In our Western mythology we're all told that we're born with a guardian angel. Yet, as children, if we tell our parents that we've seen our angel and this spirit has told us something important, we're usually told by our parents that it was only our imagination, or it was only a dream, or it wasn't real. Since we believe and trust in our parents as they are the first bearers of truth in our lives, the angels become *unreal* and we very quickly lose our ability to perceive them.

In indigenous cultures, people believe they are born with an animal spirit guardian instead of an angel. And, if you meet your personal animal spirit as a child, and speak with it, perhaps dance with it in a dream or vision, and see the world through its eyes, you're told you have received a precious gift, that you have powerful medicine, and that you should foster the relationship with your dream ally. In native cultures this natural ability is fostered rather than rejected.

Our dreams are just as real as our everyday world, we're just not used to describing them as such. Or conversely, our everyday world is just as real as our dreams. It only depends on your perception! But what do dreams, even if they are real and a precursor to our world, have to do with our lives? As John Perkins was taught by the shamans of Ecuador, to change our lives and our world, we only need to change the dream. He discusses this concept in detail in his book, *The World Is As You Dream It*, and, along with it, the importance of taking responsibility for the world we dream. To imply that we dream our reality, and that we can focus and control our dreaming attention means that we have to *take responsibility* for our lives and our worlds. *They are our creation.*

We create with every thought, with every action, with every dream. It's only once we have taken responsibility for who and what we are, and taken responsibility for the lives we have created for ourselves, that we can begin the journey toward wholeness. Only after we accept the fact that we are creative beings, that the divine creative Source is within each of us, and that whatever our circumstances are, we have created them, can we step into the path of Living in Vibrancy, experience The Glow of Being Alive, and meander effortlessly, fulfilled and in harmony and balance within the self-actualized state described by Abraham Maslow.

We have chosen everything in our lives. We have chosen exactly who and what we are. We have made this choice at every point in our lives, and will continue to choose everything in our lives right down to the very last detail. This idea is hard to accept, especially if you were born into not so nice circumstances. Or perhaps have a serious illness. Or maybe a companion you love has left you. Or you were seriously hurt in an accident. This idea of having chosen these kinds of circumstances is a bitter pill to swallow. Naturally you say, "I didn't choose that. Why would I choose something that is causing me so much pain? How could I have chosen to be born into a family with an abusive father or an alcoholic mother?" You chose it. You chose it at a level that is deeper than we have ever been taught exists, and one that our normal consciousness rarely touches. But whatever the situation or circumstance, it has been chosen. It has been precisely picked. And it has not been chosen by some punitive deity exacting punishment on us for our sins. Each situation, circumstance, and event in our lives has been chosen by us! We are beings that do nothing but make choices. We make choices, create, and manifest those choices.

Unfortunately, most of our choices are by default. We make some choices at a very deep level that we have not been taught exists or taught how to access. And others we agree to by passively becoming part of the consensual and never actively choosing. In making these choices we never ask, "Why?" In fact, we're taught by our culture and our educational system not to ask, "Why?" And when we do find the supreme courage it takes to step out of the consensual and ask, we're usually chastised, ridiculed, told we're crazy and that we shouldn't think for ourselves, and to get back into the fold. How many times have you been told, "That's just the way it is." How many times have you said this to your children? We will examine both types of choices, those made at a deep level, and those made by default, as we walk The Steps to Vibrancy.

To Live in Vibrancy you have to take responsibility for all of your choices–those made at a deep level, and those made by default. The exercises in this chapter will guide you to the place where you can know, and know viscerally–within your body and the deepest part of your beingness–that you have chosen everything in your life. You have created the life that you're living. Once you feel and truly know that you have chosen, you will be empowered to choose differently.

Sometimes knowing that you've chosen something bad for yourself kindles the big "G," **Guilt**. There's no reason for this. First, as we'll see, there is no bad or good. There only is what is. Bad and good are judgments, and we will learn how to step out of judgments. Second, very frequently because of societal and cultural conditioning and programming, you had no choice–the choice was made for you–so, why feel guilty?

Some traditions would argue that our lives are predetermined. They suggest that something called *karma* dictates who and what we are, and that living our lives is like watching a movie where our part, our script has already been written. It's true, our lives are like watching a movie, ***but we are the scriptwriters, the dreamers, and we are writing the script and dreaming the dream as we live!***

Who Am I?

Who am I? This simple question has been asked by countless people, for countless generations, for countless millennia. It reaches back in time to the first being who was aware enough to see their own reflection in a deep, placid pool of water, and point and ask, "Who is that?" To take responsibility for *who you are*, you need to know *who you are*. Yet knowing *who you are* is a task which has eluded all of us except the grandest mystics and seers. Rather than directly seeking the essence of, "Who am I?" it's better to approach the question from slightly askew. It's helpful to first define, *"Who I am not?"* Then, knowing who you are not, sneak up to the creative spark of divinity we all carry within the subtlest reaches of our hearts.

Experience

You are going to make a list, the "Who am I?" list. Begin the list with ten things that you are. Start with the most basic. I am a son. I am a daughter. I am a father. I am a mother. I am a wife, a husband, a lover, a companion. I am a (whatever you do for a living). I am a cross country skier. Don't make it a struggle to deliver the items from your unconscious to the page. Rather, let the exercise be a ceremony, a free flow from the dream world alive within you to the reality of white paper and black ink in front of you. There is no right and no wrong. Whatever comes into your mind is valid. Even if the thought seems strange, doesn't make sense, and it's not something that you generally identify yourself with, if it came into your consciousness, then it's alive within you for some reason. Write it down.

Once you have ten items, return to the first one and sit with it. Meditate with it. All of the exercises in this book are meditations, and this means opening your awareness and widening the apertures of your perception. For instance, if the first item on your list is spouse, see what being a spouse entails. What duties does it carry? What responsibilities do you take on being a spouse? What is it that defines being a spouse for you? Draw a picture of your world with yourself as a spouse, and what being a spouse means to you. Surround yourself with all of the ideas and thoughts that identify the concept of spouse to you and draw lines, threads of light connecting them with you.

Then, change your perception. Change the metaphor you are using to relate to yourself. Instead of identifying with *being a spouse*, identify with the *role of spouse*. Instead of being a spouse, let spouse be a part that you're playing in the screenplay of your life. Where did the script come from? Who wrote the part? Where did the description of the role of spouse come from? Why did you try out for the part? Did you understand the role before you picked it? Most importantly, why did you choose the role? Instead of seeing yourself *as a spouse*, see yourself as *playing the part of a spouse*. You're the actor in your own drama of life. How did you come upon that role? You weren't born a spouse, somewhere along the way you auditioned, were picked, and chose the role. Take responsibility for having chosen the part.

Once you've finished with the first item, proceed through the same steps with each of the ten items on the list. Work with each item until you can identify with it as a role in the screenplay of your life, not as what or who you are.

As you finish with each item cross it off of the "Who am I?" list, and place it on a separate sheet under a heading such as: "Things I am not," or "Roles that I play," or "Who I am not."

Once you're done with the first ten items and you see that they're roles you've chosen rather than things you are, make another "Who am I" list of ten items. Again, let the list be an easy, free flow of consciousness from the inside out. These new items will become less basic. Let the items reflect anything that you do or identify with: hobbies, jobs, educational degrees, things you do, likes, dislikes, everything and anything.

Ten items listed, work through the list in the same fashion as the first. Change your perception and see each thing, not as the essence of you, but as a role in the screenplay of your life. And remember, it's a role you are writing for yourself as you live your life.

After the second list of ten things has been transformed into ten more, "Things I am not," repeat the process again. As you work with each list of ten items let the items become more abstract. Move from the concrete, I am a husband, or mother, or bridge player, to the more abstract: I am a seeker of truth, I am a lover of knowledge, I am a creator of beauty.

As you move further and further into the abstract you will see the essence of the actor, the true "Who I am" become manifest. You will clearly reach the place beyond roles. Open your eyes and meet the writer, the creator of the screenplay of your life. Introduce yourself. Greet the essence of you. Say, "Hello."

My Life, My Choice

We are beings who make decisions. We are always in the process of making a decision. Just reading this book, working through these thoughts, and seeking knowledge within these exercises and processes is a decision you made. The book may have come to you on the recommendation of a friend, or the title caught your attention, or you liked the artwork on the cover. However you came to be reading these words and examining these concepts, it was a decision you made. Everything in our lives works that way. Everything you have done, become, tried, failed, and experienced has been a decision you made. No one is blown around haphazardly like a falling leaf in the wind. That's so important it bears repeating. No one is blown about haphazardly like a falling leaf in the wind. We choose, have always chosen, and will always choose what current we ride.

To take responsibility for ourselves, our situations, and our lives means we need to realize that we have chosen what we are. We need to know that we have decided to be in whatever place we are in our lives. In fact, we have chosen our current birth situation. Ask anyone who works in the field of past life regression. We chose our parents. We chose our families. We chose, before birth, who we were going to be in this life. A detailed look at the past life experience is beyond the scope of this book, however, we will come back to the concept of past lives with an illuminating exercise later in this chapter. For now, let's concentrate on our present life, it's the one we're currently working with.

Experience

Get a blank sheet of white paper. Make it as large of a piece as you can, poster board size is preferable. Draw yourself in the middle. Don't worry about being artistic. A stick figure or symbol will do, but make the representation something that you really feel represents you. Now think back to a major decision you made in your life. Pick a choice you made, but one you don't really feel you had a choice about. Something where it seemed as if some options were so unpalatable that there were no options, and you **had** to pick the one you did. On the diagram surround yourself with all of the options which were available to you regarding that decision, palatable or not, including the one that you chose. Put small circles around them. Connect yourself to the choice you made with a line. Next, draw a large circle around the whole lot–yourself and all of the possible choices. Now, in small circles surrounding the largest one which contains you and your choices, put all of the influences that determined your decision, and place arrows pointing from them to the large circle. Include every concern, no matter how large or small, that affected your choice.

Now, with everything in plain site, look at the influences which affected your decision–the small circles pointing to the large one. Where did those influences come from? Who put them there? Did they materialize by themselves, or did you choose them in some way, shape, or form? How did you, consciously or unconsciously, bring them into your field? See how the influences themselves were of your own choosing, and understand that you chose to be influenced by them. The influences may have been there, but you didn't have to be affected by them! One by one work with the influences and see where they came from, and why, (they're there for a reason) you put them there. Then, after you understand the origin and nature of a particular influence, cross it out. Go through the same process with each influence. Once you realize that you've chosen the influences to be there, that you brought them into your field, you can choose that they not be there.

Now, without any outside influences, go back to the original decision and choice. How does the decision you made measure up without any influences? What choice would you have made without any of the influences you pulled into your field? Why didn't you make that choice?

Now, take yourself to the next empowering step. Take the original situation and decision, and choose differently. Use a new piece of paper. Put yourself in the middle again. Write out a different choice than the one you made previously, connect yourself to it with a line, and put a circle around you and your choice. Now, using arrows connect yourself and that choice with all of the possible outcomes from that choice. Don't place judgment on anything. Without bias or thought just list all of the possibilities. List every single possible outcome that you can imagine occurring from that choice. As you proceed don't look at the options and outcomes as only possibilities. They are all **choices** under your direct control. Remember, you are the screenwriter, and when writing a screenplay, **anything** is possible.

Now, without any influences, worries, or concerns, decide which path, which choice you want to manifest. It's really that simple. We certainly haven't been taught it's that simple, but it is. When we're in a state where there are no conflicting thoughts, emotions, or influences, we manifest the choices we make. Actually, we always manifest the choices we make, we just don't realize that what we are getting is of our own choosing. The real trick is getting rid of the conflicting influences, and part of this is taking responsibility for the fact that we choose to have those conflicting influences in our lives.

Decide which path on the diagram you've made is the one you want. Cross out all of the others. Now sit with it. Envision yourself on that path and see where it takes you. Write out and commit to the paper where it takes you. More importantly for this exercise, see what influences and concerns come up that prevent you from following that decision. As they come up, examine them, see why they're there, understand why you bring them into your field, then choose them not to be there. Do this until you have a clear path to your goal.

Continue this process, but in a slightly different manner. Make a list of choices you've made in your life. Start with five or ten things. Pick one of them and using arrows, diagram out the steps to where that original choice has taken you. As an example take marriage. Married→kids→house→job→and so forth. Don't skip any steps or details. When you look back at a particular decision line, you will see that everything along the particular line which brought you to where you are now was of your choosing. As you make these decision lines with other choices you will begin to see that everything that's happened in your life was a consequence of a choice that you made. Take responsibility for your choices, and if you desire, choose differently.

The intent here is to see that you are not, never have been, and never will be a leaf blown across the landscape of your life by an unseen, uncontrollable wind. There are no unseen forces which direct our lives against our control. Everything you have ever done was your choice. Everything you have become was your choice. Everything that has ever happened to you was your choice. And, most importantly, everything you will ever do or become is your choice. Only once you take responsibility for your choices can you begin to redirect your life in the direction you want it to go. And the directions we can choose to guide our lives are only limited by our imaginations.

A Responsible Day

When stepping back and examining our lives as a whole, it's relatively easy to take responsibility for the decisions and choices we've made, and also for the outcomes we've gotten. We're able to change our focus and broaden our perception, and see that the choices we've made are ours and nobody else's. On a day to day, minute by minute basis, it's not quite as easy to see this happening. Yet the same principles apply. We choose. We decide. We affect everything that happens to us. From the puppy peeing on the carpet, to the train making us late for a meeting, to an argument with a companion–we choose. We choose everything that happens to us, and around us.

Looking at our lives this way brings up some paradoxical questions. The foremost one is, "Why do things happen to me that don't seem to fit my goals?" That is, say you're trying to get a promotion at work and everything you do to foster your supervisor's attention and engage their support fails. Are these *signs* that you're not on the appropriate path and an indication that you should be putting your energies elsewhere? If these *signs* are indeed your choice, why are you choosing them when they are counter to your stated goal? The question is valid, multifaceted, and answerable at many levels.

One level of the query involves internal conflict, and we are going to address this later in the chapter. At its most basic level, the question can be stated, "Is there a path I should be on, or, can I choose my path?" The answer is: Yes, there is a path that each of us should be on, one that is just right for us. It's a path that when we're on it we're in sync with everything–ourselves, our being, and our world. It's our unique path, the one Joseph Campbell would say, "When you're on it, doors will open where you never imagined there were doors before, and those doors are doors that wouldn't have opened for anyone else." Yes, the right path for you is waiting for you. But, and this is a big but, and it's the key, *you choose your path*. Like the screenwriter, you write it as you go. You choose! You choose! You choose! Nothing is predetermined.

So what about the blocks we stumble over? What about the hurdles that seem to be put in our way? Do we really put them there? Yes! We choose them. We place them in our path. When I speak of we, I am referring to what writers and speakers commonly refer to as our higher self, the God within, our souls, or our inner voice. This part of ourselves has been given many names and many concepts have been attributed to it. And rightly so, because this part of ourselves, our true essence, transcends anything that our linear programmed, 2+2=4 minds can comprehend. For the purpose of our discussions in this book, our higher self is that part of ourselves that is beyond our ego, subconscious, conscious, super ego, id, shadow, all of that. It is the part that is not only connected to the universal Source, but it *is* the universal Source. It *is* the divine creative potential within each of us. And *being* the creative potential entails a great deal of responsibility.

So back to the question, why do stumbling blocks occur? Why do we choose them to be there? We choose them to be in our lives as road marks. We create them as signs to tell ourselves that something is out of balance. They are messages from our higher selves, our essence, to our everyday selves that a particular path isn't right for us. And it isn't that this particular path is not right for us because it is wrong, there really is no right or wrong–an important point we will explore in depth later. The particular path where the stumbling blocks keep occurring isn't right for us because we have *not truly chosen it.* Our intent for that course of action isn't pure. Our focus, attention, and will for that particular path isn't unbending. The stumbling blocks occur when we're not committed to a particular path at a *one hundred percent, visceral, this is where I'm going, no questions, doubts, there are no back doors,* level. Two examples should help to illustrate this point.

The Hopi Snake Dance is an annual ceremony in which the Hopi pay homage and respect to the rattle snakes with whom they share the land. Through a majestic, regal ritual and community festival they seek balance with the serpents in order to avoid injuries during the year. The dancers, dressed in the finest ceremonial attire, enter a trance state through sacred drumming, chanting, and movement. Once in the trance state, the dancers handle the snakes which have been collected and brought into the arena with them. They pick up the serpents and move with them. They dance with the snakes and let the venomous creatures coil around their bodies. The dancers will even go so far as to bring the snake's head into their mouths, a move that to outsiders is the epitome of craziness in an already absurd ceremony.

The underlying theme of the snake dance is one of intent, and intention. The dancers rarely get bitten. They entirely soak themselves within the ritual and ceremony, and then release the snakes back to the land after having fostered an understanding and achieved a balance. Because of the dancer's intent–their focus, their decision and choice not to be bitten–and their one hundred percent knowing that they won't get bitten, they don't get bitten. They choose the path. The dancers step outside of the consensual and beyond our normal understanding of rattlesnakes, and *choose not to be bitten*. It's their choice, their intent, their pure purpose and knowingness that keeps them alive.

Occasionally, however, a dancer is bitten. One man, bitten, simply stated that he was bitten because his intent wasn't pure. He did not enter into the ceremony *free of doubt* and with unbending intent and pure purpose. He realized this, accepted it, even embraced it, and chose to let the natural course of events take place. He allowed himself to succumb to the venom and passed on. This dancer took ultimate responsibility for his decision to enter into the dance.

Now one might ask, "Was it his choice to get bitten and subsequently die? Was it his decision at a soul level to have his whole life turn out the way it did? Was it his choice to die as part of the snake dance?" These are heady questions, best answered in an intimate discussion with close friends over a glass of fine Cabernet. (The answers are there, and, of course, they are your choice.) Let's look at a less complicated illustration, one from my own life.

During the later half of 1997, themes and understandings of unconditional love were entering my life very frequently. These are themes and processes which are still coalescing and will eventually be the topic of a forthcoming book. It was Christmas Eve and I was celebrating with my parents. I am divorced and my ex-wife, who lives about 15 minutes from my parents, was supposed to have dropped my daughter at their house. I had picked my father up and taken him to visit my grandfather who was confined to his house because of health reasons. We were arriving back at my parent's house, and as we pulled into the drive, the garage door was going up. My mother was angry. My ex-wife had called and asked why no one had picked up my daughter yet. The signals had gotten crossed somewhere. She had expected my mother to pick her up, and my mother had expected her to be dropped off. My mother was not happy to be going out, and even less happy because a large snow storm had blown into the area, and within an hour, we had an inch of snow on the ground.

I calmly assured my mother that everything was all right, and that I would just go and pick up Alyssa. My mother agreed, and still somewhat upset, went back inside. My father followed her and I began on my way to pick up my daughter.

Now Alyssa's mother and I are not on exactly good terms, the nature of which would also be illustrative, but not exactly within the focus of this book. Anyway, given the themes of unconditional love I had been working with, I believe I should have been thinking, "This is a good opportunity to practice what I've been being taught. Wish her love and a happy holiday." Instead, I clearly remember having the sarcastic thought, accompanied, I'm certain, by a mischievous glint in my eye, "Seeing me will sure make her holiday happy." I remember this thought very clearly. I had the thought just before the car, turning off of the main road where I was waiting to make a left turn, and standing perfectly still, skidded on the icy street and slid right into the side of my car. Now, there are no coincidences. You've heard this from many writers. I had not been in an accident in over ten years.

No one was hurt. We traded information and filled out the police report. Both cars were drivable, but all of the hassles of being in a collision were set in motion. The other driver took responsibility for the collision and his insurance paid to fix my car. And I took responsibility for my part of the collision. What, you ask, was my responsibility? I was just stopped, minding my own business. What was my part of it?

I brought the collision into my sphere, into my field of existence. I created the event (originally, in writing this, I used the phrase *unfortunate event*, but that signifies judgment, and that's not appropriate) as a sign that I had stepped off the path I had chosen, the path of working with and attempting to embody the notion of unconditional love. My intent to be on a particular path was not pure, and I created, or pulled the event into my field to tell me so. I chose the collision as a sign to myself that I had strayed. I manifested it as a sign that I needed more focus in what I had chosen to embody. I was forced to take responsibility for both, choosing to be on a path, one of unconditional love, and for deviating from that path.

Please notice, and this is important, that I have refrained from using the word accident to describe the collision. Being in *an accident* implies that we are the leaf in the wind, blown around at the whim of unseen forces beyond our control. The notion of accident implies that things just happen for no reason at all. There is no such thing as an accident. The phrase *accidents happen* is an oxymoron. Nothing, absolutely nothing happens without a reason. Nothing happens without a choice behind it. To use the notion of accident suggests relinquishing responsibility, something we are all very good at doing. There are no accidents, no coincidences. We choose, and we have to assume responsibility for our choices.

How can you see this working in your own life on a daily basis? The process requires introspection, journaling, and keen, unbiased observation. Be certain that this particular technique becomes clear to you because we're going to expand on it later.

Experience

Pick a day, any day, and carry a small notebook with you at all times. At the beginning of the day make a conscious decision that you are going to record everything that happens to you. And I mean everything. This includes events and situations that you might ordinarily classify as good or bad. We are trying to achieve a non-judgmental state, so the things you write down should be large and small events, major and minor. Anything and everything should be included, but avoid placing judgment on the events. Everything should be included in an unbiased manner. An abridged sample list might include: *Made the coffee stronger than usual. Got up too late to have breakfast. Ran out of toothpaste. Looked just perfect in what I am wearing to work today. Traffic really light today. Staff at office in a strange mood. Clerk at the gas station commented on my attitude. Received a card from Bill who I haven't spoken to in months.* You get the idea. Make note of events and details, small and big. Even consider why you picked the particular day that you did for this exercise.

In the evening, in a quiet, private, secure place where you can reflect on the events of that day, undisturbed, work with the list. Take each event and see WHY it occurred. There are no accidents, coincidences, or random occurrences. Everything that happens to us occurs for a reason. And the reason something occurs is the reason we chose to create the event and bring it into our field. All of these exercises are exercises in meditation and introspection. They are all vehicles to move past the outer ego self to the inner self that creates. This is The Self that makes the world we inhabit. Work with each event and find the reason that it happened. There is always a reason we choose something, it's only a matter of looking deep enough. See why you chose each event. Why did you create a particular occurrence at a particular time and point in your life? What are you trying to tell yourself? See that you chose each occurrence for a reason.

Simple examples might include: You chose to receive a letter from an old friend because you need to rekindle the friendship, or there's unfinished business in that relationship and it's time to complete it, or you have the need and desire to comfort someone and the person who sent the letter needs comforting, or perhaps it's you who needs the comfort and help, but you can't ask for it so you are projecting your needs into another situation to be a sign for yourself. You chose the train to make you late for the meeting because your heart wasn't in it, or you weren't prepared, or you're not committed to what you're doing, or perhaps you have a need to make a grand entrance.

Let your intuition guide you as you're looking for the reasons behind the choices. Allow the reasons to surface. Don't discount anything, and don't judge. There is no good or bad, there is only what is. If you don't like the reason behind the choice that's okay. Own it. Take responsibility for it and let it teach and instruct you about yourself. Then, only after you have taken responsibility for the choice, release it and choose differently.

After you've made your way through the events of the day and have an understanding as to why you chose them, look at the list as a whole and see how the events are related. Realize how A is connected to B, or to F, and how one choice sets up and leads to other situations and choices. Take the events and map them out on another piece of paper with lines and arrows connecting them. Become a cartographer and create the map of your day. Maybe running out of toothpaste forced you to stop at the store which allowed you to run into someone who you haven't seen in months, and they just talked to a friend of theirs who is looking to hire someone for a job that would be perfect for you. See how choosing to turn onto one road led to other roads. Look at what other off ramps were available and why you chose not to take them. And look at why you chose to take the exits you did.

You can take this a step further. Superimpose this map with the maps of your life that you created in the previous exercises. How do they fit together? Why do you keep choosing the same exits? Why do you choose to be in the mountains, when you would rather be on the plains? If you're thirsty, why not drive towards a lake instead of circling in the desert?

Change the metaphor and see your days and your life as a journey. Let it be an adventure that you have created. Look at the road map you've followed and can now visualize. With this map you can accept responsibility for where you are now. You drove there. And now, map in hand, you can decide and choose exactly where you want to go.

The Past & Past Lives
Haven't I done this before?

It's difficult to discuss taking responsibility for decisions and life choices without touching upon the notion of past lives. Experts in the field of past lives tell us that the choices we make in this life are influenced by, and are in fact made because of experiences we've had and choices we've made in past lives. The shamanic traditions tell us that templates for our behaviors are carried within our luminous field, or luminous body. The luminous body is the energetic, egg-shaped bubble that surrounds our physical body. Shamans explain that these templates are carried from lifetime to lifetime, and until we recognize and release them we keep repeating the same behaviors. The circumstances of our different lives may change, but the behaviors remain the same until the underlying template, or energy is shifted.

This is illustrated by a recent healing session I performed with a man in his thirties. His primary problem revolved around a relationship, and a sense that he couldn't be, and didn't deserve to be loved. Themes of loneliness, aloneness, and abandonment were also very apparent as we talked. This problem had caused prior relationships to end, and was putting a great strain on him and his current companion.

During our healing journey he found himself looking at a newborn baby. The scene was very frightening to him, but he heard a voice (as clear as if someone was standing next to him as he describes it), tell him to enter the scene, and that everything would be all right. The voice told him that it was where he needed to be.

He allowed himself to become the baby. It was himself in a past incarnation. As a baby he was crying to be held and to be loved, but he heard his mother telling him she wasn't going to hold him. He heard her saying that he didn't deserve to be held. He wasn't alone as the baby, he was surrounded by spirits, by luminous beings, but because he was in physical form, he longed for a physical touch. He longed for his mother's touch, which he couldn't have. As we went deeper into the experience and the life of the baby, we discovered his birth was unplanned, the seventh child of the young wife of a farmer. It wasn't that she didn't love him, she couldn't love him. She was tired, overworked, and overburdened. She didn't want him, and she didn't have the energy to care for him. She didn't hate him, but she couldn't love him.

We worked with the energy, the momentum of this experience which had been carried into his current life. We healed the past trauma by releasing the energy associated with it and allowing him to feel and understand why he wasn't loved then, that he was worthy of love now, and that love was available to him whenever and wherever he needed or wanted it. As we integrated the experience afterwards many things fell into place for him: He could understand why he had a mother in this life who was extremely loving and had difficulty letting go. (The opposite of his mother in his past life.) He could see why he had difficulties in relationships in this lifetime. He could even understand why he never liked the country provincial style of furniture.

Two days after our session, his companion of two years left him a letter expressing her concerns about their relationship. He had not spoken to her about what transpired in the session before he received the letter. In the letter, his companion said she didn't understand why it seemed that he felt he couldn't be, and didn't deserve to be loved. He had never expressed his feelings about these issues to her. Their relationship changed drastically after releasing the energy of the past life, and to this day they are doing very well together. There truly are no coincidences, and we are all connected in a web of life and consciousness that goes deeper than we have ever imagined!

All of us, in the right circumstances, will have a past life experience. Skeptics to the notion of past lives would argue that it is simply our psyches or unconscious creating the experience. They would say that we never really *lived* those experiences. Whether or not we really lived those lives in the same manner we are living this one is not germane. The fact is, those experiences, memories, ideas, and emotions, and their associated energies are alive within us. They are part of us, and they are constantly influencing us–sometimes subtly, and sometimes not so subtly. And until we choose to address them, to take responsibility for them, they will continue to live in us and influence our life and lives.

While deep past life regressions are best done with the aid of someone experienced in guiding people into these realms, we can all very easily enter the energies and worlds of the past lives that live within us. Once there, we can choose to release those energies that no longer serve us.

Experience

You need a quiet place to lie or sit where you won't be disturbed. Phones and pagers should be turned off. The light should be subdued. You may want a bandanna, scarf, or eye mask to cover your eyes. You will also need some type of soothing meditation music. Reiki healing music, new age instrumentals, classical, or any subtle, relaxing and soothing music which has the effect of carrying you beyond the world you are used to will work. A drum beat, especially a monotone, rhythmic drum beat, is excellent for this type of journey.

Before you turn on the music and get comfortable, you need to decide which past life you want to visit. The past life suggestion should be open ended. It should not take the form of, "I want to see when I lived in ancient Rome", or, "I want to see when I was a queen in Egypt." The suggestion should be something along the lines of, "I want to visit the past life when I was in my power, doing exactly what I was supposed to be doing. When I was in synchronicity." Other examples are:

"I desire to visit the past life where I suffered the most."

"I desire to visit the past life when I performed my greatest good (or my worst evil)."

"I desire to visit the past life where I chose correctly (or chose wrongly)."

"I desire to visit the past life that has affected this life the most."

"I desire to visit the past life which has lessons for me to recognize for this life."

"I desire to visit the past life where I made the most mistakes." (But understand that there are really no true mistakes.)

"I desire to see what promises I made in the past that are affecting my current life."

"I desire to visit the past life where I lived my dreams."

"I desire to visit the past life where I served (or didn't serve) others."

"I desire to visit the past life where I made the same mistakes (choices) as in this life."

"I desire to visit the past life which can show me how to live this one better."

"I desire to visit the past life which is affecting a particular situation in this life." (You state the situation.)

You get the idea. Your intent should be open ended and not confined to a particular place, time frame, or situation. The purpose of your experience should be for exploration, learning, and evolution, not for merely sightseeing.

Turn the music on, put yourself in a comfortable position, and cover your eyes. Allow yourself to relax. Give yourself permission to relax, and give yourself permission to embark on the journey. If you need to, state out loud, "I, Mary Smith, give myself permission to relax, to be guided by the music and my intent, and to explore." If you are used to working with spirit guides call them. Ask them to come be with you. If you aren't familiar with your guides, it's all right, your intent will be enough.

Now, relaxed, comfortable, flowing with the music or drum beat in your very personal, sacred space, embody the decision you've made about which past life to visit. Bring it fully into your awareness and let it guide you. Say it out loud. State it very loud and forceful, as if your life depended on it.

With your intent focused and set, and your desire voiced out loud, allow yourself to journey. Let the experience unfold around you: Your experience may be visual and continuous, just like a lucid dream, or even like your waking life. Or it may be snapshots and scenes of people and places. Or it may be mostly feelings and sensations. They are all valid. The most important thing is to be one hundred percent present for the experience. Allow the energy of the experience and journey to guide and teach you.

Once you've finished, and you will know when you're done, bring yourself back to the here and now slowly. Move your feet. Stretch you arms. Take time to record the experience in a journal. Record a narrative in your own words on tape. Use crayons, colored pencils, markers, or maybe lipstick (use your imagination and be free), and draw a picture of the experience. As you write, draw, or speak more of the experience will come to you. Take time to reflect on the past life and the information you obtained. What knowledge did you receive? How does it link to the behaviors and experiences and choices in your current life? What lessons are there for you?

And most important: What did you do in the past, and in the present, that you need to take responsibility for?

By journeying and experiencing your past lives you can release the energy associated with them–if you choose. And that's critical, you have to want to release the energy and change. Through experiencing and recognizing what lives within you, as past lives, you can understand, then diffuse the momentum they are giving to your current life. By releasing their energy and diffusing their momentum you can release the hold they have on you, and step into the current life of your choice.

As you become more familiar with the technique the past life experiences you have will become more real. As the experiences become clearer you can dialogue with the people in your past lives, including the *yous* that you meet. Going back to the past to change the present or future is not just the stuff of science fiction movies. It's a technique used by shamans and medicine people from cultures across the world. As you become more familiar with the past, and your awareness within the experiences increases, talk to the *yous* you meet. Talk to the other people who have been part of your lives. Renegotiate the agreements you made that are affecting you now. Clarify promises that were not clear, and are not in your best interest now. (More about this later.) Release those *yous* and other people from the past that cling to you, and give love to those *yous* that didn't receive love in the past.

Visiting the past is not only about releasing things which no longer serve you. You can, and you should, learn from the *yous* that you meet in your past. We are truly our own best teachers. The *yous* you have been in other lives can not only teach you about what to release, but can teach you how to bring the empowering assets and attributes they have had into your current life. Allow your past *yous* to teach you how to be the *you* who *you* want to be.

Take responsibility for the present by taking responsibility for the past. Change the present by choosing differently in the past. It's your choice, only yours.

Conflict

Taking responsibility for ourselves, our lives, and our choices is not exceedingly difficult when we examine our life journey from within ourselves. Nor is it difficult when we step back a few paces and view our lives from the vantage point of an impartial observer. We have all selected our lives and it doesn't matter whether our choices and decisions were made based on cultural conditioning, our own internal desires, or external influences. The bottom line is realizing that whatever choices we've made, and this is the key, *choices we've made*, are our choices. Before we can release the choices we've made and empower ourselves to make different choices, we have to own the choices we've already made. We have to accept at a most basic, visceral, energetic level, responsibility for what we've selected.

Sometimes it will seem that no matter what we do and regardless of how hard we try, it's impossible to take responsibility. In some instances, regardless of how we examine a situation and a choice, we cannot chose differently. We seem to accept responsibility for the decisions we've made, yet we cannot chose differently. An example of this would be what we call an addiction. For the purposes of this discussion we will restrict our definition of addiction to exclude those behaviors that have a physical component, such as smoking and drug use which have large physical components, as well as alcohol abuse. (These behaviors with a physical component are still a matter of choice and taking responsibility, however, because of the physical component the discussion of them is best left for another time in order not to complicate this illustration.) Addictions for this discussion will include behaviors like always choosing the same type of companions or lovers, people who don't serve us, but we always fall into a relationship with. Or always playing the same role in the victim, abuser, rescuer triangle. Or always playing the same role with a family member, like strict parental figure, an adult child, or submissive child to a parent. Or perhaps you try and choose the promotion in your job, or the next step for growth in your business, and it just won't happen. Or you want to choose to show your love for a companion and you can't.

In many cases like these there is an underlying, unseen, unconscious, but by no means inactive, **conflict** which is preventing the new choice. By conflict I mean an underlying dis-harmony which results from stepping into the situation the new choice will bring. This is because the new choice will lead you into some facet of the situation which does not resonate with a part of your inner self.

An example of this type of internal conflict is choosing a new job or accepting a promotion. You've examined the situation from all angles and it seems wonderful, just perfect–more money, more prestige, a chance to be doing something more in line with your goals. You've discussed the change with your family, and everything is in the open–all of the cards are on the table. Yet you cannot make the decision. You cannot accept the job or promotion. Or, you know you want the job, but you can never get yourself in a position where it's offered to you. By looking for the conflict within, you will gain extremely valuable insights about yourself and your true wants and desires. Through understanding your internal conflicts you will empower yourself to take responsibility and release those choices and ideas that no longer serve you, and make the decisions and choices that will usher you into who you want to be.

Experience

Place yourself in the situation you cannot seem to attain. Make the choice you cannot make. Visualize yourself in that new job, or new house, or with that new companion. Go beyond visualizing it. Be there, in the situation. Close your eyes and *feel* yourself in whatever the situation is you desire. Feel what it's like to be in that new job, or new house, or with that new companion, and make a list of what emotions the situation kindles within you. Write down any emotions and sensations that migrate into your body. Some of these emotions and sensations will be pleasant and you will like them. Others will not be comfortable for you and you will dislike them. The ones that make you uncomfortable are the ones directing you to the underlying conflict. And the conflict is what is preventing you from attaining your goal.

Allow the subtle sensations to migrate to the surface of your consciousness. As the sensations arise, comfortable or not, pick a word to describe them, and write it down. Additionally, list how your life will change. Write out everything that will change and be different in your life. Don't spend a great deal of time making the list, give yourself a limit of five or ten minutes. This is not an intellectual exercise. It's not an exercise for the thinking part of ourselves. It's an exercise for the intuitive, feeling, and all knowing part of ourselves with which we've lost touch.

Once you have the list, slowly work with each item. Start with the first emotion or feeling. Where does it come from? Why is it so strong? Why is it there in the first place? Meditate with the feeling and see where it lives in your body. Where do you hold it? What does it tell you? What is the meaning underlying it? For the emotions or feelings which make you uncomfortable, the most important question to ask is: What is the conflict that gives rise to sensation? Do the same with all of the emotions, and all of the other items on the list. Use your body's kinesthetic sense to discover what is a conflict, and what is not. (The next section explains kinesthetic sense in detail.)

The following are examples of things which have come up with people I've worked with to illustrate how this works. You desire to live in a big house and surround yourself with beauty. There's nothing wrong with that. You have the talent and means to provide yourself those things, yet no matter what you do, you can't. The underlying conflict could be that you don't feel deserving enough to have those things. Maybe you don't feel yourself worthy. Or you may feel that if you have those things others won't. At some level you can't understand why there are *haves* and *have nots* in the world.

Or perhaps you can't make a choice of commitment to a loved one. You love the other person dearly, freely, without bound, but you can't make the choice to commit to them. The conflict may be that you're already committed to a path in life, or what you see as a mission, and being with this other person will sidetrack you. Or maybe you don't really love without bound like you think. Or you've *seen* what happens to relationships after people commit to each other, and you don't want to fall into what you think is a trap.

Another example is taking a particular job. The job is perfect for you, right in line with what you like to do, and the money and prestige, things important to you, are there. But you just can't do it. The conflict could be that the job is going to add structure to your life when you prefer to work in an unstructured, more freewheeling environment. Or perhaps the job really isn't in line with who you are, or who you want to be. Or at some level you feel that you are being seduced by things that really aren't important to you.

Just identifying the conflict within yourself is frequently enough to take responsibility for it, release it, and empower yourself to make the choice you want. Understand that conflicts arise out of judgments we impose on ourselves, and judgments which we allow others to impose upon us. Likewise, we should never impose our judgment and what we feel is correct for ourselves onto others. Another way of saying this is: Stay out of other people's business. Take a moment and think about how much time you spend thinking about what other people are doing, and judging them. A lot of time. When we do this, not only are we wasting energy, but we are really placing judgment on ourselves, because what we see in others is a direct reflection of what's within ourselves.

Everybody is responsible for **only** their own decisions. We only need to take responsibility for our own choices.

My Body Knows

Our bodies have a kinesthetic memory. This kinesthetic memory is an internal sense and knowing which can be used as a guide. Another way of saying this is that our bodies know when we are in balance and harmony, and when we, and it, are out of balance. Phrases such as, "Your body knows what's right or wrong for it," are not appropriate. In the medicine traditions there is no ultimate right or wrong. Those are only judgments we place on things and events as a result of the world of duality we inhabit. There are only behaviors and choices that serve us, guide us, and help us move toward what we desire to be and who we're becoming, and those behaviors that do not serve us–those that do not guide us to where we want to go. We've already seen what the Sufi poet Rumi so eloquently said about this. "Out beyond our ideas of right doing and wrong doing," he begins, "there is a field. I'll meet you there."

To say there is no right or wrong does not imply there are things we shouldn't do. There are actions and ideas that are right or wrong for us, but not because they are inherently right or wrong. They should only be called right or wrong because they either do or do not serve who we are, or who we want to be. There is nothing inherently right or wrong about anything.

Our bodies can guide us in choosing. Our bodies can inform us regarding an appropriate decision or choice when we can't seem to make it. The following exercise can be used as an aid or adjunct to any of the exercises in this book, or in general when you are trying to make a decision that seems difficult. Before using this technique to make a decision, it is necessary to become familiar with it, and get to know your own body and its kinesthetic sense. Despite what we may think, most of us are not wholly aware of, or intimately familiar with, our own body.

Experience

Lie down in a quiet room where you won't be disturbed. Shut off the phones. Dim the lights. You should have on loose fitting, comfortable clothing, or nothing at all. (Remember, we're in The Garden. Your body is a perfect manifestation of creation and nothing to be ashamed of!) Allow your body to relax as you allow your attention to focus on your breathing. Do not try to control your breathing. Let your breaths be natural, easy inhalations and exhalations. Once you are comfortable and relaxed, and your breaths are easy, rhythmic, and effortless, in your mind, bring yourself to a place, or into a situation, that you know is good for you–one that in your heart of hearts you know is a place of balance for you. It could be the park you played in as a child, or the woods you walk in now. It may be in the company of a favorite pet, or the arms of a loved one. Any situation that you know from the depths of your being is good for you will work. It should be a situation that brings you to a place of harmony, joy, and peace.

Once you are in this place, engulfed in the feeling, surrounded by the goodness it holds for you, scan your body. This means letting your awareness drift from part to part. Start at your feet. How do they feel? What do your toes feel like? What's their position? Their temperature? Move you awareness up your legs. How do your calves feel? Any tension? Are they flat against the ground? Move your attention up a little. How about your thighs? Are they relaxed, supple, or tense? What's going on in your pelvis? How does your abdomen feel? Is it soft or hard? Are there any sensations in your chest? How is your heart beating? What's your heart's rate and rhythm? How about your breaths? Are they shallow or deep? Labored or easy? Your shoulders and neck? What about the muscles in your face? How does your scalp feel?

Allow your awareness to methodically move through your entire body, and become conscious of your body's sensations. Take your time. There's no rush. This is a slow process of awareness, attention, and perception. Through this process you will also learn that you are not your body, but that your body is a container and a vehicle for your consciousness. Understand, and truly recognize what your body feels like in a harmonious, balanced state of being. In a sense you are stepping out of your body and allowing your consciousness to be an observer of its container.

Once you have a good sense of your body in this perfect, harmonious, balanced state, move from the balancing situation to one that you know throws you out of balance. Take yourself into a place or situation that you know in your heart is not good for you. This situation should be one that throws you off balance every time you are in it. It may be with a supervisor with whom you just don't resonate. Or maybe it's performing a task that you despise. Why you feel the way you do in the particular situation is not important at this point. In a certain sense, even places that throw us off balance are not bad because they have something to teach us by virtue of examining why they throw us off. But learning from them is not the purpose of the exercise at this time. We just want to be in a place that doesn't make us feel good.

Bring yourself to that place or situation and surround yourself with it. Be a part of it, and let it be a part of your body. Now rescan your body. How do the muscles feel? What is your body's position? How did your body's position change? What happened to your heart beat and breathing? How does your skin feel? Become aware of what your body has to tell you when it's in a situation that throws it out of balance.

Practice this exercise a number of times over a two-to-three-week period until you are comfortable with recognizing and understanding the differences in your body. Once you are satisfied that you have a good sense of how your body behaves, and that you are in sync with yourself, you are ready to use your body's kinesthetic sense to make decisions.

To use your kinesthetic sense to make a decision, put yourself in a quiet, comfortable place just as before. Let your body relax and become comfortable. Now take yourself into the situation or the decision you want to work with. In the beginning, it should be a decision that you are ambivalent about. One that you think you can go either way with, but you just can't decide. Bring yourself to one of the places you're wondering about. Put yourself into one of the situations you are trying to decide if you should venture into in *real life*, and see how your body feels. Does it feel the same as it did when you knew you were in a good place? Or does it feel like it did when you were in a bad place? If you're trying to decide between two alternatives, put yourself in both outcomes. See which your body tells you is right or wrong for you at the moment. (The use of the words right and wrong are unfortunate idioms of our language which are difficult to totally exclude.)

As with any technique you'll need to work with this one and come to trust it. To use it, you need to experience that it works and gives you the proper guidance. It's a matter of turning your beliefs into knowledge through experience. This is an important concept we will discuss in depth as we walk The Steps to Vibrancy.

Use the technique for smaller, less life altering decisions at first. Should you go to a particular restaurant with a particular companion? Should you take the kids to this place or that? Experiment with these smaller things and see that events and situations turn out the way your kinesthetic sense indicates. See what happens if you do something your body tells you that you shouldn't. Experience that the technique works. Once you've experienced that the technique works, it's time to use it for the grander, larger decisions you need to make.

You can use a corollary to this technique, which I alluded to earlier, as a springboard to further self-growth and knowledge. When a situation or event is indicated as dead wrong for you, and it causes you extreme disharmony, anxiety, and uncomfortable emotions, examine the situation through your new lenses of perception, and without judgment, and see and understand why it makes you so out of balance. Use any of the techniques in this book. Look for the conflict within you that is kindled by the situation. Why does it cause you such dis-harmony?

This doesn't necessarily imply that you should resolve the particular conflict so you can do the very thing that your body is telling you shouldn't. But with the understanding of yourself comes knowledge, and that knowledge leads to power. And power means empowerment over yourself and your life. Empowerment allows you to take responsibility for who and what you are, and become who you want to be.

Fear, Change, & Judgment

No teachings on self-understanding and empowerment would be complete without a few words on the big three: Fear, Change, and Judgment. A whole book could be written on only these three simple words, and, in fact, many books have been written about them because they are such overriding factors influencing our lives. In this section we will briefly look at them in the context of Living The Steps to Vibrancy.

Fear, change, and judgment are three of the big stumbling blocks we face on our journeys of self-awareness, growth, and empowerment. The three feed each other, resonate with each other, and support each other. They form a triangle which we are placed in the middle of from our birth, and we're not given any of the tools we need to step out of this place. This triangle imprisons us within a consensual world of struggle, inadequacy, and lack.

Our world, and the universe are filled with abundance. They overflow with abundance. By stepping out of the triangle formed by fear, change, and judgment we can realize the abundance of the world, and the *vibrancy* of our own lives.

Fear

Fear is the motivating force in our lives. We are afraid of not having enough. We are afraid of change. And we are afraid of judgment. (Although we rarely miss the opportunity to pass our judgment on others.) We are afraid of loss, and very often afraid of losing something we haven't even obtained yet! We're afraid of just about everything.

Where does this overwhelming fear come from? And, how do we get it under control? Our fears, like the vast majority of our behaviors, are learned. Our fears are given to us as part of the enculturation process. And this enculturation process begins very early in our lives.

My medical background is in Obstetrics and I delivered babies for nine years. About 6 months before I left private practice I participated in a particularly beautiful delivery. It was textbook. The baby came out pink and crying. Mom had a short, uneventful, and uncomplicated labor. Dad was there and supportive. And it was at nine in the morning, not three. Well, as soon as the baby delivered it was obvious that it was a big baby. Its red cheeks were pudgy, and it was just plain heavy. I handed the baby off to the nurse and told dad to go see his son while I finished what I had to do. Dad walked over and watched the nurse dry off the baby and put him on the scale to be weighed. It was a digital scale with big red numbers. The nurse placed the baby on the scale, the numbers went blank, then returned.

The baby weights nine and a half pounds. It's a big boy. Now, this kid isn't even a minute old, and the first words it hears out of its father's mouth are, "Wow! You're a big boy. You're going to grow up and be a football player! Aren't you!"

We become tied into our culture and belief systems very, very, early in our lives, and probably before we're even born because there is little doubt these days that we're conscious and learning when we're *in utero*. As we grow and become part of our culture and society we learn about them and rapidly acquire their traits. This is strikingly apparent if we open our eyes and look at other peoples without judgment or fear–without the concept of *the other*.

In our culture it is considered rude to belch after a meal. We consider it a disgusting sign of disrespect and a lack of control of our bodily functions. Yet in some oriental cultures, belching after a meal is a compliment, a sure sign that you liked the food, and a signal of respect to the host or hostess. In fact, the louder the belch the better. If you don't belch, it's a sign of disrespect and impoliteness.

This is a seemingly trivial example, but through it, and the baby story, we can see how we're taught right and wrong, acceptable and not acceptable, and that this teaching begins very early in our lives. It is less trivial when it's a matter a racial prejudice and social persecution. And fear is no different from either of the two examples we have just looked at. We're taught to fear what is different from ourselves. We're taught to fear not having enough. We're taught to horde because someday we won't have anything for ourselves. How many of us were enculturated and programmed with the phrase, "You'd better save up for a rainy day." That's a slap in the face to the abundance around us. But if these fears are learned behaviors, how do we step out of the triangle and unlearn them?

Working through The Steps to Vibrancy and exercises in this book is a way to relinquish fears. By Living The Steps to Vibrancy you can retrain and reprogram yourself through experiences, and learn that fear is not something you need or have to have in your life. When you live with fear, you get fear. When you live without fear, you have nothing to fear, because fear just doesn't enter your life. This is one of the ways the notion of karma is explained–you get what you are, or have been. It sounds simplistic, and, in fact, it is. It's very simple, but we haven't been taught this.

Fear is not a natural state for us. It's not a natural state for any animal. Look at nature. Animals do not live in a constant state of fear. And whether we want to admit it or not, we are animals by virtue of our biology. We are part of nature. And nature is part of us. Animals exist in a natural, relaxed state of calm awareness and readiness. I had the pleasure of visiting the Galapagos Islands a few years ago. There is no fear among the animals there. When you walk on the islands, you're accepted as part of the terrain. You are welcomed as part of the nature that exists there. When you walk on the islands with the animals you are back in, and part of, the garden. Certainly the fight or flight phenomena exists. If an animal is threatened it quickly moves into a heightened state of readiness and awareness, but it doesn't perpetually live in this state like many of us.

Experience

Use the preceding exercise, My Body Knows, but instead of dis-harmony, substitute fear or a fearful situation. See how your body feels. Then see where that fear lives. Look and see what part of your body holds that fear. Instead of looking for the underlying conflict, examine the underlying fear within a situation or decision. What is the fear which drives that choice or lack of choice? See where that fear comes from. Look for and understand when and where that fear was placed into your consciousness. "You're going to be a football player," may have been "You're never going to amount to anything," or, "It's a cruel world out there." Most importantly, look back and see where the fear has come up in your life, and see that no matter how significant the fear was, you came through the situation unscathed. You're reading this book now, aren't you?

Change

We hate change. Most people despise change. When we examine the greatest causes of stress in our lives, all of the stressors involve change. Change of jobs. Change of companions (divorce). Change of living situations. Death of a loved one (change of support group). And yet there is nothing, absolutely nothing in our world or our lives that doesn't change. Nothing gives us that constant, unyielding security which we all strive for. Absolutely nothing is permanent. Actually, there is one constant, one everlasting, unchanging thing–the Source of everything to which we are all connected. But we don't believe it, and we don't know how to realize it in the context of our lives.

We change every second, but don't know it. You've changed in just the past few seconds by reading this paragraph. Reading these concepts has changed you. The change may be big or small, but you've changed by virtue of reading and considering these words.

Everything changes because without change there is only stasis and stagnation. Without change there is no growth, newness, or evolution. In fact, if there were no change, none of us would be here. Something had to change in order for us to exist. Life is a dynamic, moving, transforming process. Life is a process, not a thing. It's a process that at its very core involves change. Without change there is no life. Without change and movement there is only stasis and stagnation–death in the sense we usually use that word.

So, how do we change the agreements we've been given? How do we go from despising to embracing and loving change?

Experience

Accept that change is the natural order of things. Look around you and see that everything changes. Go for a walk in the woods. Nothing is stagnant. Everything is changing. Drive into a city or town you're not familiar with. Everything is in flux. Nothing is standing still. Life is bubbling all around. Look at old and new pictures of the same place–it's different. Look at old and recent pictures of yourself. You've changed. Change your perception and see the movement, not the stasis, around and within you. Accept that nothing, including yourself, is static. See that change is the natural order of things. Change makes us uneasy because of fear. Fear of the unknown.

Use the exercise for taking responsibility for decisions, My Life, My Choice, earlier in this chapter, but instead of a decision, work with a major change in your life. Diagram it out. See that changes which have happened in the past have not led to the dire consequences you imagined. See that, in fact, most of the major changes in your life have turned out well. Add up all of the time and energy you expended worrying about and fearing the change. How could you have better used that time and energy?

We worry about change because we fear things going from good to bad. Well, as we've discussed, there is no good or bad, there just is, and every situation has a lesson for us, an opportunity, and a way to grow. But even if we accept that things are good or bad, everything changes! Good goes to bad, and bad goes to good. We certainly don't despise a change that we feel is in our benefit and taking us someplace we judge as better!

Your body knows that change is not bad. In fact, your body is changing every second. Only about one percent of the cells of your body and their constituents are the same as a year ago. *Only one percent.* You truly are not the same person you were a day ago! When faced with a change, use your body's kinesthetic sense that we just explored to *feel* that the change is all right. Know that it's okay with, and within, your body. If you get an indication that the change does not resonate with your body, use that as a springboard to understand why. What is the fear or emotional conflict associated with the change? Use it as a grand opportunity of self-growth. Learn about yourself. With knowledge comes power. Any change we can contemplate pales against the greatest change of all–our death. (We are going to learn this later as we walk The Steps to Vibrancy when we meet our personal death.)

Judgment

We spend a large portion of our time categorizing things. This is not necessarily bad or wrong, because if we didn't, we wouldn't be able to communicate with one another. If we didn't all categorize the essence of a tree as the same thing, we couldn't talk about a tree. However, a great amount of our time is spent placing things into the categories of good or bad, and right or wrong. We spend the majority of our time looking for, and creating absolutes where there are none. Everything is relative, and right and wrong are part of the world of duality we have stepped into in order to learn, play, and experience.

We can use the example given earlier about belching after dinner to illustrate the point. In one culture it is very acceptable and right, and in another culture it is very unacceptable and wrong. Where's the absolute? The predominant religion in the United States tells us it's wrong to engage in sex before marriage, yet our mass media programming tells us it's right. And, in other cultures it is right to experience many partners before marriage. Many of our religious traditions tell us killing is a sin, yet they proceed to qualify this by saying that it's okay to kill someone in certain situations, as in a war, or in the name of *our God*. We are even honored for how many we've killed. We pass judgment all of the time where no judgment should be passed, because there is no absolute right or wrong.

In the shamanic traditions, as seen in all of the great spiritual traditions when separated from their cultural milieu, there is no inherent or absolute right or wrong. There is no absolute, autonomous good or evil which exists independently in the universe. There is no independent right or wrong. There is only what we create and pass judgment on. There are only those situations and energies that serve us and carry us into who we are becoming and who we want to be, and those that don't. Simply put, some things serve us, others don't. But this does not imply right or wrong. What serves one person may not serve another. What may serve us at one time, may not at another.

As we've seen, the basis of the great spiritual traditions is a universal oneness, and not only a connection with the Source, but the very identification of that Source within everything, and every being, including each of us. The statement that God is in, and in fact is everything, and everything is in God, echoes clearly throughout the world's spiritual quests. And everything means everything: good and bad, right and wrong, ugly and beautiful. Remember the East Indian mystic who was asked about Brahman. "If all is Brahman, if all is the Divine radiance, how do we say no to filth and ignorance and prejudice?" His answer was, "We say, yes!" We embrace everything, because *every thing* is creation. Everything is Brahman, or God, or Buddha stuff, or the Christ Light.

Experience

Make a vow, for just one day, to go through that day without passing judgment on anything. DO NOT classify anything as good or bad. DO NOT judge anything, or anyone, as right or wrong. (As we've said earlier, when we judge, we are really judging that part in others which is a reflection of what's within ourselves.) See events and situations you come across as things that either serve you or do not serve you. See how they may or may not serve another person. Be totally and completely nonjudgmental about everything you see, every situation you find yourself in, and every situation you observe someone else in.

Look, without judgment, at why you have chosen to bring particular events or situations into the field of your life. We choose everything in our lives. And to understand ourselves and our choices we must step beyond judgment. You may have chosen to bring the worst thing imaginable into your life, but that thing could be the very situation you needed to propel yourself into who you are becoming, and who you want to be.

We have to embrace it all in order to find the vibrancy within ourselves. We have to be able to say "yes" to the beauty in everything. And to embrace it all, we have to put ourselves aside, and step beyond judgment.

Play, Play, Play
Why are we so serious?

Despite the serious sounding title of this chapter, *Take Responsibility*, it's not meant to be serious. In fact, it's not supposed to be serious at all. Taking responsibility, and life in general, is not supposed to be taken seriously at all. Life is supposed to be fun! We're here, in this magnificent world, to play in the field of time and space, and celebrate life. We're not here to suffer, self-indulge, and pity ourselves. We're here to play, learn, and experience. And we had better do just that, to the fullest, because our time here is very, very short.

Why do we take everything so seriously and forget to play? Because we are victims of our enculturation. We do what we're told. Like lemmings following each other to the water, we act the way we've been taught to act without ever examining the agreements we've been given. Taking life so seriously and forgetting to play is something we've been taught. It's an idea about life we've been given and just accepted without any consideration. And this seriousness we carry around deep within our bellies is not a natural state for us. Use the kinesthetic body exercise and see that this is true.

How do we release this idea? How do we relinquish our seriousness? How do we renegotiate the agreement and learn to play? One of my teachers' teachers used to tell him, "It all begins with the children. What we teach them. And what they can teach us." This simple, elegant statement may be the biggest truth in this whole book. Everything begins with the children.

Experience

Spend time with children–preferably those younger than seven or eight, which is when our adult prejudices begin overriding the power of their innocence. Spend time with them and look at the world through their eyes. Experience how they have no past or future, but are always alive in the present, the eternal now. (More about this in Step Into The Empty Space.)

And children know. They know about those things that can be can be known, but not spoken. We only need to listen. I was recently visiting my parents. My nephew, Paulie, and niece, Amanda, were there. Paulie is five years old and Amanda four. My mother has been through a great deal of stress in the last few years, much of it because of a world-view she has not been able to release. We were having dinner and she commented that all she wanted was peace. Not world peace, but peace in her life. Paulie was sitting next to her. None of us were aware that he was listening to our conversation. After she made her comment, Paulie blurts out, in a voice that didn't even sound like his, "You have peace!" He smiled sheepishly and went back to eating. The comment went by unnoticed by the other people at the table. For me it was sage wisdom.

"You have peace!" Everyone who is reading this book has peace. We all have peace. It's only a matter of perception. And children have the perception which we search for everywhere. They have what we look for everywhere except within ourselves. The innocence we all have as children is our power. And it is real power. It is the power to be anything and do anything because nobody has told us we can't. Nobody has informed us of any limitations. And when we're not taught we have limitations, we don't have any. None whatsoever.

Allow children to give you the gift of innocence and play. Talk to them about their *friends*. Ask them about their *imaginary friends*, the companions we all had as children until we were told by adults, *who know better*, that they aren't real. Ask the children about their friends, and remember yours. Remember the connection to grace you had as a child. Remember the beauty your friends brought into your life. Then call them back. Let your seriousness and heaviness drain away through the connection to the beautiful, magical, and real world of a child.

And give the children a gift in return. Allow them to retain the beauty and power we all come into this world with. Don't make them relinquish what they will spend the rest of their lives searching for–that powerful inner essence which is directly connected to the same Source that creates stars, and informs sunflowers how to arrange themselves and look towards the sun. We all want the best for our children, and we shouldn't put our children in the position of having to read this book.

Children know how to *live in vibrancy*. We lose our childhood much too early. We are born as children, vibrant, complete, whole, and in beauty. We should live and pass on in the same state.

People often ask, "What about the rest of the world?" They say, "If I live like a child, in innocence and beauty, what about the world around me? It's still contaminated by filth, squalor, and prejudice." The answer is very simple. The universe is very, very accommodating. In fact, the reason it is so accommodating is because we create it. The world is an idea. It is a dream. And the way to change the world is by changing our ideas of it, and of ourselves.

When we change our agreements and ideas, we change our perceptions. When we release the hold our preconceived notions have on us, we change. And when we change, our world changes with us. Don't worry about everything and everybody else. Everybody is responsible for their own world. Everybody can change themselves and their world if they desire. You are only responsible for taking responsibility of yourself.

Change yourself, dream your dreams, and allow the life you desire to embrace you. It's your choice.

TWO

Get Into Your Power

The privilege of a lifetime is being who you are.
Joseph Campbell

HAVING TAKEN RESPONSIBILITY FOR WHO we are and who we have been, we are now ready to find out who we should be. Olga Kharitidi, M.D. in her book *Entering the Circle*, a vivid and stirring account of her initiation into the world of Siberian Shamans, describes their belief that there are only seven types of Spirit Twins, or things that we can be. These are Healer, Magus, Teacher, Messenger, Protector, Warrior, and

Executioner (someone who makes things happen, not someone who kills).

Ancient traditions from around the globe, as well as contemporary spiritual teachings all allude to our soul's purpose. They all suggest that we incarnate into a particular existence, and into a specific life situation and set of circumstances for a special purpose. We enter into the field of time and space at a unique place and time to learn certain lessons, to experience certain powers, and to manifest and use certain talents. We all have a special talent we are supremely good at, and that talent is our power. Our power is that special gift we are supposed to be experiencing in our lives. It's what Joseph Campbell calls our bliss. It's that thing which brings us joy beyond belief, and when we are in our bliss, following our unique path, we are always where we should be, doing what we ought to be doing.

In the shamanic traditions, this is echoed by the belief that for medicine people, synchronicity and serendipity become operating principles in their lives. There are no chance occurrences, the universe conspires on their behalf, and struggle melts away. We might understand this idea by saying that we should make our hobby what we do for a living, then we are never working. With this perception, the idea of vacations to *get away from it all* melts away, because going on vacation means we feel the need to escape from what we're doing, and so we're probably not doing what we love to be doing!

We all have a path we ought to be following, a special talent we should be manifesting and utilizing in some way. This is a unique journey, our own hero's journey where synchronicity and serendipity become our operating principles. Following our bliss, and being on our own path requires that we step outside of the cultural conditioning and paradigms which have been imposed on us and live from our hearts, not our heads. An example is the young girl who excels in art, but is told by her family that she will never be able to make a living being an artist. So instead of following her bliss and finding her own personal, unique happiness, she becomes, perhaps, an accountant, and is never able to bring her passion into her life. She then lives an inauthentic life of drudgery, existing in what T. S. Eliot so aptly calls the Wasteland, always trying to find the one missing piece. It's amazing what we do to our children, and it's the same story over and over. Imagine how less rich the world would be if Mozart had been told, "Listen, Amadeus, it's tough to put food on the table as a composer." Or maybe that's what he was told, and he stepped past it and followed his bliss.

Another problem we run into is *they*. My grandfather recently passed away and my mother inherited some money. She and my father have always enjoyed traveling, but have not been able to go anywhere the last 5 years because of her father's health. During a conversation at dinner one evening, I suggested they take the time and experience just how varied and magnificent our garden is by taking a trip around the world. My mother's eyes lit up when I said this. Then she returned from a brief moment of bliss and commented that, "*They* say you shouldn't make any fast decisions at a time like this."

Who are *they*? I have no idea who *they* are. I do know that we spend a great deal of time and energy making decisions for other people. I know that daily, most of us give up our own power and don't take responsibility by allowing other people, *they*, to make decisions for us. And I most certainly know that your first spontaneous thought, your first idea about what is right for you, is **always** the right choice. It's only once our minds push away our intuitive side and we begin listening to *they* that we lose sight of what's right for us.

This chapter will guide you into remembering your bliss, that special passion, unique to you, and only you. It will empower you to step outside the bounds of your cultural conditioning and past the misguided wisdom of *they*, to follow your personal bliss. The exercises will take you to a magnificent place of wholeness and balance so that when it's time to pass on you can look back at your life and instead of wondering where the time went and feeling that you were passed by, you will be able to say, "I haven't missed anything. I lived the life I was supposed to have lived, being who I was supposed to have been."

How Do I Know I Have A Power?

Accepting that we all have a special talent we should be exercising in this life is the first step to finding your power. This special talent has been called many things by many people. Words or phrases like life's purpose, soul's purpose, mission, and special talent can all be substituted. I like the word power, but in this context, power does not mean what we usually think it does.

Power for us generally means having control over someone or something, and it usually suggests domination. In the context I'm using it here, power means a connection to Source. It means being informed by Source as our guide in life. It means connecting with that which we have chosen to be doing. In native cultures someone who is power–full, filled with power, is strongly connected to Source. They are in touch with the transcendent. This connection could manifest as a lucid dreamer, an intuitive, a ceremonialist who can make it rain, or a healer. Someone who is power–filled is someone who knows that each of us is filled with creative potential and can manifest their unique potential to create. Our power is our unique connection to the Source of everything. And we all have a special talent or power.

I can't give you logical proof that you have a power, a special talent which puts you in synchronicity with yourself and the world at large. It's something that evades our rationality. But once you've done the exercises in this chapter you will know that you have a power, and what it is. You will know it because you will have experienced it. Actually, you already know what your power is, it's really only a matter of remembering. Once you know your power the rest of The Steps to Vibrancy will teach you how not to give away your power any longer.

Struggle verses Effort

Before we begin exploring our power, a distinction needs to be made between struggle and effort. They both require what we call work, but one is a hardship, the other is a joy. Most of us are taught that life is a struggle and that we have to suffer through hardships to obtain the things that we desire. Where this belief and perception of the world came from is not important, although the third chapter of Genesis immediately comes to mind when we ask this question. Whether this belief is true or not is not important. What is important is that it's only true if we make it true. Remember, when you change your perception, you change the world. What is important is that when we are doing something we dislike, something that doesn't resonate with our true selves, we struggle. When we are in our power, doing what we're supposed to be doing and following our bliss we may still be *working hard*, putting a lot of time and energy into the task, but we are not struggling. We may be putting all of the effort we can into our work, but if it brings us joy beyond belief and makes time stop, we're not struggling.

A classic example where struggle and effort are apparent is the workaholic. We all know someone who we consider a workaholic–someone who seems addicted to their job. Someone who works what we consider ungodly hours and sacrifices all of their time. The question is: Are they struggling? Or are they applying effort? Are they unhappy, or are they in their bliss? Are they doing what they do for monetary reasons, or is it their passion, their power? Do we call them workaholics with the usual derogatory overtone because we think they are hurting themselves through the struggle, or are we envious because we're not in our power? Are we jealous of them because we're not following our bliss, and they are? Do we wish we could be living our passion in our daily lives? We can!

This distinction between struggle and effort is important, and I want to be certain that the difference is clear. We can look at many examples from other people's lives, but it's our own lives that we want to explore.

Experience

Think back to when you were in school. Remember when you were in high school, college, or graduate school, it doesn't matter. Now, what was the subject you hated? The one you disliked with a passion. The class that no matter how much time and work you put into the subject you just couldn't get it. For me, it was the math of advanced physics, differential equations and all that stuff. I could spend hours with the formulas and not understand them. It was an immense struggle for me. Remember your problem subject, then remember what struggle was. Use the kinesthetic sense that you developed in the previous chapter. How does your body feel when you're engaged in a struggle? Do you want to live life like that?

Now remember the class you loved. The material that simply flowed for you. The class that you enjoyed so much that you spent extra time with the subject. The one you wanted to take a second time. How does your body feel in that place? In the first instance you were struggling, in the second, applying effort.

What activities do you struggle with now? What do you spend a great deal of time doing where every moment is a struggle? Is it something you consider a chore like mowing the lawn or changing the cat litter? Is it your job? What are your hobbies? What can you spend nights until two or three in the morning doing without getting tired? This is effort.

We can live our lives struggling doing things we dislike, or we can spend our lives, in our power, applying effort. One is infinitely more satisfying than the other. It's simply a choice.

When I Grow Up
I Want To Be A....

We all wanted to be something as we were growing up. And this thing, whatever it was, is something very special to us. We all had some special dream, and we all knew what it was. And we all lost touch with this special something when we reached the stage where we were told, "You need to have a secure job and career," or, "You'll never make a living at being a...." (You finish the sentence.) What we are doing with The Steps to Vibrancy is creating a life, the one we forgot we were supposed to have. Living then follows naturally.

Experience 1

Go to your sacred space. Turn off the phones. Burn incense. Light candles. Dim the lights. Put on some soothing, relaxing background music. Do whatever relaxes you, brings you to a place of peace and comfort, and creates an area of subtlety where miraculous changes can occur. Next, let yourself drift back to when you were younger. Return back to the time and place before your innocence was lost and dreams were as real as the floor or chair you're sitting on. Give yourself permission, if only for a small amount of time, to be young and naive again. Breathe in the simplicities of your childhood and let the memories blanket you.

What did you enjoy doing? What did you want to be when you got older? Who did you admire? (In or outside of your family) Did you love watching the figure skaters in the Olympics? Did you marvel at your grandmother tending her garden? Did you relish watching your father put on his uniform?

Let the images and memories flow freely and jot them down on a piece of paper. Let the emotions flow too. Laugh as you remember your parents. Cry as you recall dreams given up. Emotions are energy, and some energies need to be unbound and released. Make the list as long or as short as it needs to be. Use your intuition. Use the knowledge of yourself that's inherent within you. Don't worry if the things on the list seem possible or not. Nothing is impossible, we have only been taught they are. (More about this in Choose Your Circle.) For now, nothing has to make sense, and nothing is impossible.

Now, list in hand, work with it. Review the items one by one. Use the kinesthetic body sense you've been developing. Which things on the list are right for your body? Which ones aren't? Again, the mind and intellect should not be playing a role here. Converse with your rational self. Tell your rational self you honor it, and that you appreciate its help and guidance, but for now you'd like it to remain quiet. And I mean really talk to it, talk to yourself out loud. Don't feel silly. Your self will listen. Don't be at all concerned if anything on the list seems reasonable or not. Don't worry if it makes sense or if it seems impossible. Allow your body to inform you what's what.

Take your time going through the list. None of the exercises in this book are a race. You've spent years not using and not honoring the parts of yourself you're now getting to know. Give yourself the gift of the time necessary to develop these new relationships.

Once you've been through the whole list, there will be a few things that stand out. If there is only one thing, you've got it. You've found your power. If there is more than one thing which feels just perfect for your body look for the thread that weaves them together. Follow the energy and find the common theme. For instance, dancing, gardening, and horseback riding may all be equal for you. Use your intuition and bodily sense to locate the common theme, the link between them. In the above example, they are all a celebration of life. They all are very kinesthetic. They all require a certain sense of freedom and expression that you may not be allowing yourself.

Now, once you have your power, either specifically or as a theme, step back, broaden your perception, and see the myriad ways in which that power can manifest in the world. As we discussed at the beginning of this chapter, the Siberian shamans believe there are only seven things that we can be. For us healer typically means a doctor. However, healer can have many manifestations. A mother who loves, cares for, and guides her child into who they are supposed to be is just as much of a healer as a true physician healer. (I say true healer because most physicians are curers, not healers. And, there is a big difference between curing and true healing.) A healer can manifest as an attorney who does arbitration, or as a CEO who treats people like people and is more concerned about employees than the bottom line. A true healer can manifest as a landscaper who treats his job as his art, or as someone like Mother Theresa.

Experience 2

Once again, step into your sacred space and allow the images of your power to flow through you. Jot down the thoughts and feelings as they arise. See how your power can become manifest in your life. Realize the myriad ways your power can unfold for you as a unique individual. If you get many images and suggestions, use your kinesthetic sense to see what's most correct for you. Again, and I can't stress this enough, leave your reason aside. Nothing has to make sense. Nothing is impossible. Forget about what *they* will tell you.

Now take this exercise one step further. Close your eyes and visualize yourself in your power. See yourself living it. Where are you? Who are your friends? Who are your associates? What is your life like? This is your life, not your living, and despite popular wisdom, your living and your life can be in sync! Get specific. What state and town are you in? Don't limit yourself. What country? Relax and allow the images to come. They will. Your life is waiting for you. It's stalking you. It's yours. It's your power. Recognize it, feel it, and take it.

My Passion My Life

While the preceding exercise is one of the most powerful for cutting through to the core of things and getting to your power and your connection to Source, there are other ways to uncover your power. We all wear different colored glasses which are altering our perceptions. What works for some people may not work for others. This exercise and the one following may guide you to where the previous one didn't. It may open doors which you didn't see when you first looked.

"Take your passion, and make it happen." These words from the late 70's movie Flashdance should resonate with each of us. We all, every one of us, have a passion. We all have something that gives us joy and comfort, purpose and connection. We all have a passion, yet very few of us make it happen. Few of us allow our passion to manifest in our lives. The passion I'm referring to is not erotic passion, although when we are engaged in activity we are passionate about we frequently feel an erotic sensation or sensual quality. This is because when we're engaged in something we're passionate about we're creating. We are manifesting the creative potential we share with Source. And sexual energy is creative energy. Sexual energy is the creative potential manifest, so it's no wonder we get an erotic buzz when we're doing something we feel passionate about. (One of the difficulties we encounter is the terrible perception we've been given about sexual energy. This perception, like most of the perceptions we've been given, needs to be altered.)

In the indigenous medicine traditions, the concept of soul retrieval is critical and is illustrative of the idea of passion. For shamans, our soul is multifaceted and individual parts of it, which are conscious, can flee because of trauma or fear. These soul parts leave and travel to someplace they consider safe. The person who has experienced trauma and soul loss frequently lives feeling incomplete and disconnected from the world and from themselves. While the problem is difficult to solve within the Western perception through which we view ourselves, the difficulty is easily addressed in the shamanic world view. The shaman simply journeys and brings the missing piece, and the energy associated with it, back to the client. In the tradition I practice I have been taught to visit four parts of my client's soul when I do a soul retrieval. One of the places I go is called the Chamber of Passions. In it, I look for that person's passions. I find what connects them to Source, and what it is that manifests their unique connection to Source in this life. I look for what embodies their creative potential.

I once worked with a man who was going through a divorce after a marriage of over 25 years. In his heart he was feeling all of the loneliness and loss which we associate with the change of a long standing relationship. After some other work and healing of old and new wounds, I did a soul retrieval for him. In the Chamber of Passions I found a man, walking by himself in a beautiful, spacious, sun drenched prairie. He was perfectly at ease and at home with himself, the nature around him, and his own thoughts and intellectualizations. His passion was his aloneness–not loneliness, but aloneness. His passion was to be with himself churning over and examining ideas and concepts. In his life he had lost sight of this passion by being extremely close–perhaps too close–with his spouse and his family. He tried to manifest this passion in his life, but failed, as evidenced by a number of unfinished manuscripts in his desk drawers. Bringing back this lost part of himself released much of the loneliness he was experiencing and gave him a new boost to finish his books.

This gentleman wrote a poem to help honor and embody the soul piece and energy that was brought back into his life. Below is the last stanza.

When I wrote that last poem

I had to look up the word hallelujah

To spell it right

And I realized

Never before in my life had I written hallelujah

And I thought to myself

Oh, the first sign that at long last I have found

That thing I have been searching for all my life–Joy

And so I say

Hallelujah!

Experience

This exercise calls for becoming still and looking to see what resides within your own Chamber of Passions. As before, go to your own personal sacred space where you are relaxed and won't be disturbed. With this exercise, as with all of the exercises in this book, feel free to call on your own spirit guides to assist you. Call on them to help you with your stated intent. In this case, your intent is to remember your passion. Even if you don't know who your guides are and have never worked with them, or you don't believe in them, try it anyway. You'll be amazed at the results. Verbalize out loud, "Guides who are here to assist me, be with me and help me to discover, understand, and realize my passion." (Or whatever the intent is of the particular exercise.)

Your intent now is to travel to that part of your soul and inner self which holds your passion. It's that place of yourself which knows your unique connection to Source and where your creativity is manifest. Remember, and then write down whatever drifts into your consciousness. The knowledge may come as visualizations, images, feelings or intuitions. Honor whatever form your experience takes. Your experience is yours, and yours alone. And whatever the experience is, it is the correct one for you. See where your images and emotions carry you. Work with the ideas and thoughts. Use your kinesthetic sense and see which ones resonate with your body, and which ones do not. See which ones stimulate you with an almost erotic passion and sexual quality. Those are your direct link to the source of your creativity.

Follow the steps in the previous exercise with the ideas that arise. Broaden your perception. See the infinite ways passion can manifest in this world. And, most importantly, see how it can manifest in your world. Don't be concerned if it seems impossible.

The word impossible doesn't exist for the shaman. Visualize yourself engaging in your passion. See your life. Who are you? Who are your friends? Where are you? Take your passion and make it happen. It's yours. It's your choice. Choose.

Myths & Metaphors
Choose the ones you want to live

Joseph Campbell used to say that reality is those myths we don't quite see through yet. We will work much more with this concept in Choose Your Circle. For now, I want to introduce the idea of how we live within a certain metaphor that we've been given, and then work on changing the metaphor in order to help us find our power. In truth, the whole of our world is an idea, an idea we've been given since birth. When we change our perception, we change the idea. And when we change the idea, we change our world.

Our lives are entirely dictated by the particular myths and metaphors we've been born into and inherited. Our Western myths include having been cast out of the garden, being separate from nature, having to struggle and toil for our food, atoning for sins we've never committed, working hard—frequently at something we hate yet we're told we have to do—until we're 65 when we can retire and enjoy the golden years, etc. These are only a few of our disempowering myths, and these are the ways we've been taught to order our world. They determine our reality. And as we've said, reality is those myths we haven't quite seen through yet. Once we've seen through them and realized they are stories we accept as true only because we've been told they are true, they will be replaced by new myths. And these new myths are inherently more beautiful, empowering, and sustaining than those we live with now.

We can never go back. We cannot go back to old myths which once served us, but now only keep us tied to a past which is gone. And the past is truly gone. We need to carry a reflection of it with us to remember where we have come from, who we have been, but we can never go back. And we ought not to be trying. We ought not to be holding so desperately onto something which is gone. We don't have to allow our past to relentlessly haunt us and keep us fixed in a place and life which we don't want. In order to evolve and step into who we are becoming and who we desire to be, we need to step into new myths, new paradigms, and new ways of ordering our world and our reality. By changing the myths we use to engage the world and assemble our reality, we can step into our power and live the life we ought to be living.

The next experience calls for changing the metaphor you use to order your life. A metaphor is a way of describing an object or idea with words or phrases that are not commonly associated with the object or idea, yet draw attention to a likeness between the common and uncommon. Instead of using the metaphor of life as a struggle, as a punishment, and as toil and strife where you have to suffer to get the things you desire, you are going to change the metaphor. You are going to look at your life as your art. Our lives are our art, though we rarely view them as such, and *art is creative potential manifest*.

Experience

View your life as your art. Look at your life as your craft and see what craftsmanship went into producing it. See what beauty and majesty you've created. We are creative beings. All we do is create. We create our world and our life every single second of every single day we're walking and breathing in this magnificent garden we call Earth.

Don't be shy, and do not be critical of yourself. And do not under any circumstances whatsoever view your life, your creation of beauty, your personal work of art and masterpiece, by anyone else's criteria. We have all created something grand, glorious, and magnificent, and the only standard we need use is our own. Remember, it's much easier to be a critic than a creator. There is no judgment here. No judgment whatsoever. And absolutely no right or wrong! A true artist creates for themselves, and for the divinity and beauty of *the act of creation*. They are not concerned with the opinions of others.

What have you created? What medium did you work in—paint, clay, stone? Are you a sculptor or a painter? What kind of brush strokes did you use? Was it a landscape? A portrait? A bust? Is it complete, or unfinished? What point are you at now? Are you just gathering the materials, or applying the last coat of glaze? Where are you stuck? Look at it from a different angle and see a different reflection. Do you need to bring in a new color? Once it's done, then what? Begin another masterpiece. Who said we're limited to one? We can live as many lives as we want!

What is your art? How did you manifest it in your life? And more importantly, how do you want to manifest it in your life now? Your life is your art. It's your choice to be an artist, a creative being in the field of time and space against the backdrops of infinity and eternity. Passion, power, and art are synonymous in this context. What's yours? It's waiting for you. It's stalking you. Take it. It's your choice. Choose.

I Know My Power! Now What?

Now you know what your power is. You've found it. It may not be what you thought it was going to be. And it certainly may not be what you wanted it to be. But you're there. You've got it. You've grabbed hold of your personal ring of power. Now what? What do you do with it? What do you do with your power? It's simple. You get into it. Do it. Get into your power. Step into your power and allow your power to manifest itself for you and within the context of your life. Allow your life to organize itself for you. The universe will conspire on your behalf and your life will self-organize if you allow it. Put in the effort, not the struggle.

Now, you might remark that this is easy to do on paper. Words are cheap, the cynic might comment, and it's easy to say, "let your life organize itself," but out in the *real world* it's not so easy. Well, what's real? *Reality is what we choose it to be.* Reality is those myths we haven't quite seen through yet. Essentially we have two options. Settle for the reality we've been given, the consensual. Or, step out of the consensual and create our own reality. Have you ever heard adults talking about a child and saying that, "They're in their own world." Well, there's nothing wrong with that. Children do live in their own worlds, and are happy in them, until we make them like us and bind them into our world. We can all live in whatever world we desire and experience whatever life we choose. We choose our realities and the universe accommodates itself to those realities.

The primary reason we have trouble getting into our power is because we make excuses why we can't. We're extremely good at making excuses and coming up with reasons why we can't do something. In fact, some people make an art of it. In an absurd way it's their power. This is such an important topic that the third Step to Vibrancy is Eliminate Excuses–a whole chapter of this book. For now we'll put the excuses aside.

To get into your power, simply, do it. Take it step by step. Large or small steps are all right, whatever size steps you are comfortable with. Just remember, there may come a time when you have to let go of the first trapeze before you see the other one. And you may have to do this even if you're not certain there's a net underneath you somewhere. Take the steps towards your power, and see your power become manifest in your life. Your power is something natural for you to be doing. Your power is what you *ought* to be doing. Imagined obstacles will melt away when you are in your power because you're on your path. Focus your intent and step into your power and the life you *ought* to be living.

For many people this will really seem like letting go of the trapeze. That's okay. That's perfectly all right. Either let go of it, or keep one hand on it. Do whatever is comfortable for you. But you have to test your power. You will never turn belief into knowledge without experience. You have to test your power and experience that it's yours. You need to experience it to own it. Take a chance and see how the unexpected enters your life. In fact, when you get into your power, the unexpected becomes the expected. The universe works. Allow it to work for you.

There's a native American story about an elder and a youngster which eloquently sums up this idea of simply doing it and taking that grand chance. A young adult coming of age is about to go out into the world. He's leaving his village and everything that he has known and has been taught is real. He's worried and anxious, and has no idea where the other trapeze is. The youngster goes to the elder of the community and asks for advice. The elder sits him down and, after an appropriate period of silence to cause just the right amount of tension in the young person, he begins speaking. The elder tells the young person, "When you go out into the world, you're going to come to a great chasm. When you get to it, you're going to look across and try desperately to see the other side. No matter how hard you try, you won't be able to. When you're at this point, right at the edge of the great abyss, and you know that you can't turn back, there's only one thing you're going to be able to do. Jump! It's not as wide as you think."

Experience 1

Talk to people who are in their power. You'll recognize them. We all know people, or know of people who seem to be in balance and in just the right place at just the right time, all of the time. Ask them about intuition and knowing and faith–whatever you call the inner sense of peace and knowingness. Ask them about the unexpected. Listen to their stories about how the greatest leaps they took were not things they had planned on or ever imagined. Allow them to tell you how synchronicities and serendipities work in their lives. Ask them about the difference between effort and struggle. They may not recognize the context you're presenting to them at first, but as you speak and explain the concepts, they'll know.

Don't be afraid to approach people who are in their power. We've already spoken about how fears hold us back and prevent us from stepping into who we want to be. People truly in their power and in synchronicity with themselves and the world relish opportunities to share their insights. When you first introduce yourself, they may not exactly understand your queries. But as you talk to them, they'll know what you're talking about.

There are abundant examples of people who have stepped out of the consensual and into their power. The American woman who moved to Peru, without forethought or planning, and became a successful herb farmer and author. The man from an upper class Jewish family from the east coast who now lives in and leads trips to Amazonia. The woman who quit her day job and now does energy work with animals, and is booked for weeks in advance. The single most important thing to realize is that *you are no different than them*. You are no different than anyone who is in their power. You are no different than anyone who you might look up to and admire, or envy. The only difference is that people who are in their power are leading the life they ought to be living, and you're not. All you have to do to be like them is **Get Into Your Power**.

You should also meet people who are doing something similar to what you have discovered is your power. Talk to them and find out about their chasm. Ask them how it felt to let go of the trapeze? When did they finally jump? Ask them how they came to the knowingness that started them on their path and got them into their power? They may be doing exactly what you think you should be doing, but remember that no matter how similar it appears, it is different. They are who they are, and you are who you are. They are on their path, and you are on yours. No matter how similar the paths appear, they are unique because you are unique. Your path is yours, and yours alone.

Someone once wrote that there are only two or three human stories, but they go on repeating themselves as fiercely as if they've never been lived before. Your story, your path, and your power is unique, no matter how many times it's been lived before, because it's yours!

Experience 2

Visualize–Visualize–Visualize!   Everyone who teaches spirituality or techniques for self-empowerment and manifesting talks about visualization. Why? Because it works. Visualization works. Visualize yourself in your power. See your life. Draw pictures. Commit to paper what you are doing and bring the life you ought to be living a step closer to the field of time and space. Draw who you're with. Make a picture of where you're living. Visualize it. See yourself in your power. Do it as a formal meditation. Do it while you're walking. Do it while you're on the bus or train. *See* yourself in your power. Meet the you who you truly are.

Take the visualization a step further. Verbalize it. Verbalize it loudly. Say it. Shout it as if your life depends on it; because it does. Singing and chanting is important to all shamans and native cultures. It is a way of calling on the spirits and voicing intent. The medicine people say that when you sing, you have to sing as if your life depends on it. Shout as if your life depends on it–and it does–the most important words of creation, "I am _____." You fill in the blank. Let the universe hear your request. Then get out of the way and allow the universe to respond.

Shamans also say that when our intent is pure, our attention focused and unclouded, our purpose clear-crystal clear, and we speak loudly, from our hearts, the spirits hear us. The spirits hear us clearly and they open doors and paths that we never imagined being available to us. We only have to take one step towards the spirits, and they will take ten steps to meet us. Let them hear you!

Get into your power. Whether they're big or small steps, just take them. The power is yours. And it's your choice. Choose.

THREE

Eliminate Excuses

> *Several excuses are always less convincing than one.*
> Aldous Huxley

THE SINGLE BIGGEST STUMBLING BLOCK we face in stepping into the life we desire and Living in Vibrancy is excuses. We spend the majority of our adult lives making up excuses for why we can't be what we want to be, why we can't have what we want to have, and why we can't do what we want to do. We view the universe as a giant ogre waiting with a raised sword ready to cut us down at every turn. The world we get is the one we expect to get. It's that simple. If we believe the world is out to get us, then it will get us. If we believe the universe is accommodating and is our ally, then that's the world we will live in. A wise person once said, "All the world's my oyster." That's true if we want it to be. Einstein, near the end of his life, was asked, "What is the most important question to answer?" This was after he had created the theories of relativity and done many of the other great things for which he is remembered. He said that the single most important question one can ask and answer is a simple one: Is the universe hostile, or benign? We live in the world we choose to live in. The universe is what we choose it to be, and when we change our perception, we change the world.

We're extremely good at creating excuses. For some of us it is our art. None of the excuses we come up with for not being able to get into our power and do what we're supposed to be doing are valid. This bears repeating. None of the excuses we come up with for not taking our power and living the life we ought to be living are valid. None of them. They are all rationales and reasons we've been given since our birth. They have been handed to us, or more accurately, thrust upon us by our families and peers, cultures and societies. The hostile universe we live in is the one we've been given. And we can choose differently.

How often do we tell our children, "You can grow up to be anything you want." Then later when they say, "I want to be an astronaut," or, "I want to be an artist," we tell them, "That's very hard," or, "Do you think you're good enough?" or, "There's no money in that." (See how we get our values.) Even worse, children are often told things like, "You'll never be able to do that," or, "You'll never amount to anything," or, "You're going to grow up to be just like_____." (Fill in the name of a family member who is not well respected.)

Our patterns for creating excuses are established very early in our lives and reinforced by our cultural stereotypes. Our media does little to help us step outside the bounds of our conditioning and eliminate the excuses holding us back. In fact, media reinforces our beliefs in our excuses. How many sitcoms reinforce the belief that one needs to follow the normal pattern–go to school, get a job, get married, have kids, retire when you're 65, and so forth. How much of our news tells us what a dangerous and hostile place the world is, and that we have to be on guard for our life every second? Just about all of our news. However, in fact, many more beautiful and loving things happen in the world every single day than all of the things we consider bad which are reported by our media. We just don't hear about the good things. How much of our advertising tells us how we have to struggle? Just about all of it. And how much advertising tells us we have to plan for the rainy day and be ready when the sword of the universe fall on us? Almost all of it. This is why the insurance industry is one of the biggest industries in the world. Having to plan so purposefully for the rainy day implies that it's going to happen. And when we expect it to happen, it eventually does. These are all perceptions we've been given. We've been given a hostile universe that we don't have to hold onto or buy into. It's simply a matter of choice.

I was recently visiting with a wonderful couple in the Midwest. The gentleman, a man in his fifties and a true seeker, showed me a book he was reading. It was written by a relatively well known African spiritual healer. Now this healer has a system and a world view that works for him. He heals people. There are documented cases. The theme of the book he wrote is protection. Everything in the book is about how to protect ourselves from the world. Why? Because he makes a statement in the first chapter of his book that the world is inherently evil. Now I don't know about you, but I choose not to live in an evil world. We get the world we think we're going to get. Simply put, whether the world is evil or not is a matter of perception and choice–nothing more. Think about how much greater of a healer this man could be if he didn't need to expend as much energy as he does protecting himself. What if he lived in a benign world and could put all of that energy into his healing?

None of the excuses we hold dear and clutch to ourselves are valid. None of them. We'll begin with the Ten Biggest Excuses. First we'll list the Ten Biggest Excuses, then review each one and understand why none of them are valid.

The Ten Biggest Excuses

1) I'm not good/worthy/deserving.

2) I'm not smart enough.

3) They won't like me.

4) I'll be alone.

5) Nobody's ever done this before.

6) It's not acceptable.

7) It's not what I'm supposed to do.

8) I don't know how.

9) It won't work.

10) But..../Maybe....

This list should not come as a surprise to anyone. We use these excuses all the time. In fact, before we go any further, stop reading and get a piece of paper and pencil. Look over the list of excuses again, and then think back to the last 24 hours of your life. How many of the Ten Biggest Excuses have you used in the past day. And, how many times have you used them? Be honest with yourself. Be painfully honest and look at how often you make up excuses to not do what you want, or ought to be doing. How many times has one of the biggest excuses just popped into your mind and you followed it along to its inevitable, disempowering climax without any thought whatsoever?

Now, as you come to the realization of how many excuses you make to not be doing what you would like to be doing, don't start feeling bad, guilty, or unworthy. Don't beat yourself up over it. (We're good at doing that too! We've honed it to a razor's edge.) There is only what is. We've been given the excuses and we've accepted them–nothing more, nothing less. They have became part of our psyches, and part of our syntax and the way we order the world by default. Once they're ingrained in us, we start believing them. And once we believe them, we're done for. Our task is to recognize this, and accept it without judgment, because without them, we wouldn't be who we are. Then, step past them into who we want to be.

To be in our power and on our path, Living in Vibrancy, we need to eliminate the excuses that keep us from being what we should be, or what we want to be. And who we should be is who we want to be. There is no difference between the two. We are creative beings and we can create ourselves in whatever image we choose. In fact, we do it all the time! We just don't recognize it.

How all of our excuses become part of our operating system is a book in itself. In the shamanic traditions, change, real change at the energetic level, happens instantly. The understanding of why things were the way they were may or may not come. We have both a rational and a mystical part, and our rational part intellectually likes to understand the why of things. Our mystical part couldn't care less about understanding; it understands at a level we will never touch with our rational selves. It helps our rational side, the part we are more in tune with, to order, categorize, and make sense of things, but that's not what's important. The change is what's important. Likewise, understanding where the excuses come from is not really important. We're given them, like whether or not it's polite to burp after a meal, as part of our membership rites in our particular culture or life. What we need to do is eliminate the excuses, period. That's what's important.

I'm not good/worthy/deserving

Simply put, this is a bunch of #$%@! We are all deserving of as much beauty, happiness, and health in our lives as we choose. But we don't choose it because we don't feel deserving and worthy of it. We are all part of the divine. We are all part of the creative source, an unlimited, infinite process from which anything and everything arises. In fact, we are all not only part of it, we are it! If we believe the Bible where it says that we were created in God's image, how can we be anything less than God?

Where does the attitude of not feeling worthy come from? We're given it like everything else in our lives. We're given it by our society and culture, family and peers. I was raised in the Catholic religion. My grandfather recently passed away and I attended the mass for his funeral. I had not been to a Catholic service in quite a long time. As I watched as both an observer and a participant I was struck by an amazing contrast. The energy of the Christ Consciousness was palpable. It was just radiant. It was beautiful and I could feel it weaving through the building and wrapping itself around me and the other people. But the attitude of the priest and congregation engaging it was frightening. The divine was right there with us. It was all around us! But neither the priest or the congregation could embrace it. They wouldn't allow it to carry them outside of themselves. Why?

The whole of the ritual was so disempowering. For me this disempowerment was summed up in the consecration of the host. The consecration is where the magic happens and the small piece of bread transforms and **becomes** the energy of the Christ Consciousness. The words as the priest was holding up the bread, which would become the body of Christ and embody the energy of the Christ Consciousness which lives within every one of us, made me cringe. As the priest held up the host he and the congregation all repeated, "Lord I am not worthy to receive you." **Lord I am not worthy to receive you!** That's what we teach our children! Repeat that every week, or every day as you're growing up and then still wonder where feelings of unworthiness and undeservingness come from.

Now you might ask things like: What about homeless people? What about people living in the street? What about people who are destitute living in squalor? People who are starving? Selling their bodies? Do these people choose these conditions? The answer may surprise you. Yes. They do choose. We all choose every single one of the situations that arise in our lives. Our problem is that we pass judgment on these situations. We pass judgment on other people all of the time, and in doing so, we judge ourselves.

We all choose. And this includes those people who are in places and situations we can't imagine being. We can't, during this life, understand their soul's journey. (We ought to be concerned with our own journey, not everyone else's.) This doesn't mean that we shouldn't offer assistance, love, support, and compassion to those people who we feel need it. But we should not pass judgment on them or their situations. And we should not be attached to their life. We have our journey, and they, like us, have theirs. This is the whole notion of compassion without attachment.

Now you might also ask, "I'm happy with myself, I feel deserving, but why can't I get what I want, or be what I want?" Many times this has to do with contracts we have made with ourselves or others which we don't realize we've made, and which domino into other contracts that we never imagined. In Quechua, the ancient language of the Inca, the word for contract is *mañay*. *Mañay* essentially means an agreement either with ourselves or with another. These contracts are very powerful and we unconsciously uphold them at all costs. The concept of a *mañay* is a bit difficult to describe, but easy to understand with an example.

I recently worked with a client who is a very pleasant woman in her thirties. We worked on her issue of worthiness. Through our session together, we discovered how she had been taught to be unworthy and undeserving. She remembers her father always using phrases like, "Oh, that's good enough," and, "You don't need that." It's even present in her life and her relationship with him now. She wanted to put a small deck on her house. His comment was, "You don't need that. It's good the way it is."

She wasn't conscious of how this had been a theme throughout her life until our healing session together. Through her life the idea that what she had was good enough and not being deserving of more became part of her syntax, her way of perceiving and engaging in the world. It was her method of organizing her reality. It was part of her energetic core and needed to be released.

The insights we achieved about how this came about as part of her relationship with her father were grand. They were a place she had never gone before, and they helped her a great deal. But we needed to work with the energy of the unworthiness. We needed to get to the core of where this whole dynamic began and release the energy and momentum of these feelings in her. The insights, without the release of energy, would have been nothing more than contemporary Western psychotherapy and would have not helped her.

The release of the energy came as part of a soul retrieval and renegotiating a *mañay*, an agreement made by her in a past life. During the soul retrieval I found a young girl and her grandmother. The grandmother was in a rocking chair knitting, and the girl of seven or eight was sitting on the floor holding the yarn. The setting was the early part of this century in a rural area. The grandmother was poor. She was extremely poor but was content in her life. She accepted what had come her way and was comfortable in her place. The little girl worshipped her grandmother. She loved her beyond belief. And, out of her love, she had promised her grandmother that she would be just like her. I heard her say it. In a tiny, little voice, she firmly and resolutely stated, "I love you grandma. I'm going to be just like you." This simple, innocuous promise transcended that life and became transformed and interpreted as not being able to have the things she wanted. The little girl promised to be just like her grandmother, and that unintentionally included not necessarily being poor, but not having the things she wanted.

During the soul retrieval I brought the grandmother and the little girl together. The grandmother clarified things for the little girl. The radiant older woman told her wide-eyed, innocent granddaughter how much she appreciated her love and adoration, but that she didn't have to be like her. She told the little girl how much she loved her, and that she could be herself and have whatever life she desired. The release of the energy associated with the *mañay* and subsequent healing have allowed miraculous changes to occur in my client's life.

Experience

First, take a deep, close look at yourself and your life. Examine yourself objectively, without judgment, and admit to yourself that many of the things you would like to have, but don't, are things that you don't feel you deserve. We're all in this boat together. We all have issues of worthiness, but they arise from a different source in each of us. Before we can release anything and shift the energy, we have to own it. Look in the mirror and admit to yourself that somewhere within the radiant being staring you in the face is churning a phrase similar to, "Lord I am not worthy to receive you." In truth, we believe we are not worthy to receive ourselves. This belief is what inhibits us from receiving the miraculous gifts the universe has for each of us.

Then, ask yourself, "Where does my unworthiness come from? Does it come from my upbringing? My family? My religion? My society?" Use your kinesthetic sense and see where the undeservingness lives within you. Follow the energetic thread and see where it leads. Let your intuition and the energy guide you and see where the unworthiness comes from. Then know that it is a *mañay*, a contract which you never consciously agreed to. Understand that it's an agreement you were given, not one that you decided on and entered into willfully. And then void it. Make a new contract with yourself. You are just as deserving as a sunflower looking up at the sky–deserving of as much light and warmth and love as it wants.

I'm not smart enough

News flash: If it's your power, the life you're supposed to be living, then you are smart enough. If your power is your destiny, then the universe will conspire on your behalf and nothing in the consensual world can prevent you from living the life you ought to be living. Every one of us is smart enough to be doing what we're supposed to be doing. Ask yourself, what does being smart mean? What is intelligence?

In our culture smartness and intelligence is the ability to perform better than someone else on standardized tests which we have arbitrarily said measure intelligence. This is one of the greatest injustices we have done to ourselves, and continue doing to our children. Smartness and intelligence have absolutely nothing to do with standards and arbitrary measures, but have to do with what our power is and what we're supposed to be doing in our lives.

We all know anecdotal stories of the physicist who can do math on par with the best supercomputers, but can't balance his checkbook. Or the chess champion who can't find his way navigating around an unfamiliar city. We all know people who excel at particular things and have certain incredible talents, but cannot do other simple things we take for granted. These people are certainly intelligent by our standards, but outside of their unique path, they fail miserably at activities others find mundane and simplistic. An Indian from the Andes may not be able to balance a checkbook, but a chemist from Chicago may not be able to weave, or herd llama. We don't need to be smart or intelligent to be in our power because our power is natural for us. Most people in their power have never had any formal training to be doing what they're doing and on standardized tests would fail miserably. I have worked with medicine people from around the world learning different techniques, yet the majority of the healing I do with my clients comes from my heart, my intuition, and from doing what I'm supposed to be doing.

Experience

Talk to people who are in their power. Seek them out and question them. Most of them will tell you that they never had any formal training that applies directly to what they're doing. Their strength comes from their intuition and inner knowing. Their strength comes from doing what they are supposed to be doing, being on the path which is just right for them, and for them alone.

Examples of people who followed their intuition, and their hearts, and stepped into their power are all around us. I personally know a successful newspaper publisher who never had any journalism training or any formal writing classes, and actually hated English in school, an advertising CEO who never had any formal advertising training, and a successful song writer and playwright who never had any formal training in either.

Being in our power is not about learning about our power, or learning techniques. Being in our power is about stepping into what is a natural talent for us. We don't have to be intelligent to breathe, it's natural for us. Likewise, we don't have to be intelligent to be in our power, it's ours. We only need to choose it.

They won't like me

Who is *they*? *They* seem to carry a lot of influence. *They* are always saying this, and *they* are always saying that. *They* are always telling us what we should and shouldn't be doing. And *they* are always telling us who we should be. But just who are *they*? Who won't like you? And, more importantly: Why do you care? This excuse is multifaceted, but underlying it are the themes of deservingness (of love), acceptance and being liked by others, and fear of change. There's also a pinch of loneliness wrapped up in the package, but we'll discuss this later.

Yes, if you step into your power, there will be people who won't like you. Even people who are close to you and say that they love you may not care for you once you're in your power. Friends, family, spouse, and peers may not like you once you're being who you want to be. They may ridicule you. They may call you crazy. They may fear you and even turn their backs on you. This is perfectly normal. People don't like, and resist change. People fear change. And, if you change, the people close to you may not understand, and they may not like the you that you have become. Everybody you know has a plan for your life and an idea of who they think you should be. People don't like people who change and step beyond who they think they should be. We've discussed the fear of change already, but mostly though, and this will never be admitted by anyone on a conscious level, those who know you may come to dislike you because of envy. They may be jealous because you are stepping into the life you're supposed to be living.

Do it. Step into your power. It's who you're supposed to be and what you're supposed to be doing. For every person who comes to disdain you and drops out of your life there will be many, many more who come into your life filled with love and beauty, and honoring you for who you are and what you're doing. This is a guarantee! I say this from personal experience, and I've worked with countless other people who have walked through a storm stepping into their power, and have come out renewed and surrounded by a beautiful social group who honor them for who they are *now*.

Experience

Look at your life now. Who are your friends and companions? Some you have known for years. Many you have only known for two, three, maybe five years. Remember your life before you knew these current people. There were others who were your close friends. Life is an ever changing flow and our friends and companions flow with us. They flow into and out of our lives. That's the way it's supposed to be. If people leave your life because they don't like you, others who do love and honor you will fill the void. How many close friends do you have? Five? Ten? Twenty? There are over 200 million people in the United States alone. It's not that difficult to imagine forming new friendships.

There will always be people who don't like you. We innately desire the acceptance of others and for others to like us, but no matter who or what we are, there will be people who don't resonate with us and our path. No matter who or what we are, there will always be people who don't like us and don't agree with what we're doing. That's their path, not yours. Life is not a popularity contest. Don't give up your power and life because of someone else and the need for their acceptance. Be on your path and in your power. Do it with love, and love will come to you.

I'll be alone

Aloneness and loneliness are two different things. We can be lonely in a crowd of a hundred thousand people if we choose to be. But we are never alone. You are not alone even if you are hiking in the middle of the Andes at 17,000 feet.

We are never alone. Life, awareness, and consciousness is bubbling everywhere. We've simply lost the ability to perceive the sensuous worlds surrounding us. We can choose to be lonely, or we can choose not to be lonely. It's a choice, no different than any other choice.

Being on our path and in our power can seem very lonely at times. This is normal. If we weren't alone on our own personal path we would be sharing someone else's path. And if it is their path, then it isn't ours. We all have a path and a power unique to us, and that unique thing cannot be shared. It's for us, and us alone.

We truly are never alone, however, being by ourselves away from familiar voices and sounds is a blessing at certain times. Like everything in life, being alone is part of a cycle. Life is a process by which its very nature is always in flux and changing. It's necessary to be by ourselves at times. It is in these times, when we are seemingly alone, that the hidden things within ourselves which need to bubble to the surface of our consciousness can do so. A powerful Eskimo shaman from the Arctic has said, "You will only hear true wisdom when you go far enough away from people so that the voices of men cannot be heard." It is in these times, when we are alone, that the truth of our own lives is given the freedom to rise to the surface of our consciousness and be heard. Without these times of aloneness, we will never taste the truth within ourselves. This truth is our truth, and our truth alone.

Experience

Two short exercises will help put this excuse to rest. First, review your life and recall times of transition, like when you moved or went away to school, changed jobs or got divorced. Remember times when your life was turned over and your social supports and peers vanished for a time. You may have been alone. And you may have been very lonely. But you came through it. New supports and peers eventually appeared. It was a transition from one life to another. We live many, many lifetimes within our single life. Also, remember what went on inside of you during these time of aloneness. How did your perception of yourself change? What things about yourself did you have to face that you needed to face? Change your perception. These times of aloneness and transition were periods of growth and renewal, not devastation.

Second, give yourself some time alone now. Make a time for yourself when you will be really alone, where you won't be disturbed, and the voices of the world can't touch you. Give yourself at least a 24 hour period where you won't have any contact with anyone. No phones. No faxes. No pagers. No radio or television. No contact whatsoever. Preferably, go to an isolated retreat center where you will be alone, with only yourself. If you can't do this, then stay at home, but make certain that everything's turned off. Many people find it uncomfortable to be with themselves in silence for even a short time like 24 hours. Try it. See what parts of yourself bubble to the surface that you were not aware of before. See what parts need to rise up and be heard. And as these parts speak, listen to them, and hear them. Hear them with your heart. Even if you don't think you can be alone for 24 hours, try it and be empowered at the end of the 24 hours by having completed something you didn't believe you ever could do.

Take yourself away from the voices of men, and listen to the sound of the universe, the heartbeat of life–your unique sound.

Nobody's ever done it before

Come on now! We use this excuse all the time, yet the ridiculousness of it has been proven over and over. Nothing that is new and innovative has ever been done before. (At least within the field of time and space we're in now.) Where in the world would we be if people like the Wright Brothers, or Galileo, or Thomas Edison said, "Nobody's ever done it before, so I don't know how in the world I'm going to." Nothing would ever change. Nothing new and innovative would ever find its way from the imaginal world to our world of time and space.

When I teach workshops, someone always asks if the experiences they are having are *real* or *just their imagination*. In truth, there is no difference. If the experience and information someone gets changes their life, then it's real. It's that simple. The imaginal world is just as real as the ordinary world we live in. It's only a matter of bringing things back from the imaginal realm and making them manifest in time and space. Think about it. Everything that's in our world, everything that we use, from our pagers to our faxes, from our cars to computers existed in someone's imagination first! Everything that is in our world was imagined by someone before it became manifest in our world. Everything! Walt Disney once said, "If you can imagine it, you can build it." The truth of this statement has been proven over and over and over.

Experience

Use your kinesthetic sense and feel within your body if what you imagine you should be doing is what you ought to be doing, then change your perception. Change your perception to: Nobody's ever done it before. Good. I'll be the first. Or, nobody's ever done it before because I'm supposed to be the one to do it first. Or, nobody's ever done it before, I don't understand why. It's so simple.

When you change your perception, you change your life. Then, you change the world.

I shouldn't, it's not acceptable

We grow up in a society and a culture learning the *shoulds* and *should nots*. However, there are no absolute shoulds or should nots. All of the shoulds and should nots we know are learned, and they are relative. We've talked about this before and used the example of burping after a meal. In the US we would never imagine doing it. In some Asian countries the louder the burp the better. As it's been so eloquently pointed out, when we mature, our task is to slay the dragon whose every scale contains a should, or a should not.

We all have our own personal dragons breathing fire across the nape of our neck at every turn. We all have buckets filled with scales upon which are written our own personal shoulds and should nots. And when we're done with our own dragon, our neighbor's dragon will be hovering over us to take its place. These dragons seem real, but they aren't. They are projections we create based on the way we've been brought up, enculturated, and taught to order our world to fit in with the reality we've been given. When we face these dragons with the sword of real perception in hand they melt away, and the truth of our unique life–our truth, our power, and our path–will take their place.

Experience

Use your kinesthetic sense and let your body slay the dragon of shoulds and should nots. Allow your body to inform you what is appropriate for you. Our only task in life is to be who we want to be, and there is no right and wrong. Who we want to be is our choice. Our choice alone. Slay the dragon, find *your truth* and be in your power. It's what you should be doing. It's the life you ought to be living.

It's not what I'm supposed to do

By whose criteria? Whose criteria do you use to determine what you're supposed to do? Your family's? Your friends'? Your culture's? Your power is generally not what you're supposed to be doing by the criteria of the consensual. And the criteria of the consensual is the criteria of your family, your friends, and your culture. What you are supposed to be doing is not what you've been told by others you're supposed to be doing. **And we all know how much others like to tell us what to do**. Your power is your power, not anyone else's. It's what you're supposed to be doing. Respectfully shield yourself from those people who tell you it's not for you, and it's not what you're supposed to be doing. Release yourself from the grip of anyone who tells you who you are supposed to be, and what you are, and are not, supposed to be doing. And in reciprocity, do not fall into the trap of telling others what they ought to be doing. Stay out of other people's business! Their life is theirs. Let them live it with all of the glories and tragedies they choose. It's their right.

Experience

Use your kinesthetic sense. Learn to trust your body and your intuition. Let your body, through its feelings and sensations, tell you what is right for you. Your body knows what you're supposed to be doing. And it's your choice. Go ahead and choose!

I don't know how

Yes, you do know how. You knew how to breathe when you were born, didn't you? Your power is no different. You know how to do it. Your power is within you. It may be a matter of learning some formalized steps in order to organize your power and place it into a framework that your reasoning and logical side can make sense of. But you already know how to do it. You know how to do it at a deep, visceral, bodily level just like you know how to breathe. And as you step into your power, the fact that you know how to do it will become obvious to you.

Experience

Whatever your power is, just try it. Do it. Experience your power. Try it on your own, or in a more formal setting. Take a class. Get a job doing it. A word of caution about formal training is warranted. I have a dear friend who is a musician. He just loves music. It's his life. It's his passion. And it's his power. And he took some formal training. He learned a great deal in the formal training, but his primary reflection is that music school made him hate music.

In the beginning we frequently need a framework in which to place our power. But your power is yours. To manifest your own unique, individual presentation of your power you eventually need to step past any existing frameworks and make your power uniquely yours.

Once you begin doing whatever your power is you will see how natural it is for you. But you need to take the first step and try. It's been said that for every step we take towards the gods, they take ten steps to meet us. It's true. And it's the same with our power. Let yourself be amazed at the innate abilities you have. They're yours.

It won't work for me

It won't work for me is all about risks. Something may or may not work for you, but how do you know if you don't try? And at the most essential and basic level, whether something will work for you or not depends on if you want it to work or not. What truly matters is if you believe, really believe with the totality of your being–your mind, heart, spirit, and soul–it will work.

There is so much old wisdom around this excuse. The first phrase that comes to mind is: "It's better to have tried and failed than not to have tried at all." While we should never regret anything, we will always regret not having tried something much more than we will regret having tried something and failing. If we don't try, then we'll never know.

If you truly think it won't work, then it won't. It's that simple. But if you know, if you know in your body, if you know with your kinesthetic sense that it's right for you, then it will work. It will work because you've chosen it to. And you will never experience that it works for you if you don't try.

Experience

Take the first step, and see how quickly an awkward walk transforms into a flowing run. You have to take the first step though. Experiment with your power. Try out your power as a job, or a hobby, or a Sunday afternoon adventure. Just give it a try. You will find how being in your power is as natural as breathing.

But..../Maybe...

You finish the sentences. You can also add, "What if...." to the list. And, add the biggest *What if*, "What if I fail?" **What if you succeed!** We live in the world we perceive, and the world we perceive is our choice. If we live as a pessimist, we get a half full world. If we live as the optimist, there is abundance beyond imagination. Within eternity anything is possible. Enough said.

These are the Ten Biggest Excuses. We are all familiar with them because we've all used them over and over. They are part of our operating system and the way we've been taught to engage the world and ourselves. And, as we've seen, none of them are valid. They are only valid if we choose them to be valid. And, **we don't have to choose any of them.**

Experience

Now, make a list of your ten biggest excuses. Don't just think about them. Write them down. Many of The Ten Biggest Excuses will resonate with you. You know that you've used them over and over. See which of The Ten Biggest are also on your ten biggest list. Then add more. Don't stop at just ten. List all of the excuses that you use. A useful format is, "I can't because...." You complete the sentence. I can't because of my spouse. I can't because of my family. I can't because of my past. I can't because of my education. You get the idea. Get all of your excuses down in writing so that you can release their energy and momentum and be done with them once and for all.

Next, after everything is in black and white, go over the excuses. Why do you think they're valid? Are your excuses valid for you because they are true, or because you've been told they are true and believed it? Are they valid because you've experienced them as true? Maybe your experience of them as true is because you've believed them to be true by default?

Broaden your perception. See your excuses against the bigger backdrop of your life. Are they really reasons not to be in your power, or are they excuses that you've accepted by default? Are they waters you've never tested because you've been told they're too cold and have never even stuck your toe in? There are no excuses for not being in your power. It's yours. Take it.

The I'm not good enough syndrome

This is such a deeply ingrained excuse that it deserves special attention. A whole book could be written on this premise, and many have. All of the books dealing with this excuse are worthwhile and I suggest finding the one that fits you, the one that resonates with you the best, and work with it. Use your kinesthetic sense and your intuition and see which spoke on the wheel to truth is right for you. This section will present insights not found elsewhere, and some powerful ways to completely eliminate this excuse.

The *I'm not good enough* excuse is a syndrome of our culture. We constantly judge ourselves by ideals and standards which have been created for us by our culture. Our mass media and advertising constantly bombards us with messages on what an ideal body is, what an ideal house is, what an ideal car is, what an ideal Sunday afternoon is, and what likes and dislikes we should have. We are ceaselessly and relentlessly told what and how we should be, yet most of us cannot, do not, and should not be living these societal ideals. The founding fathers of this country were very perceptive when they suggested "life, liberty, and the pursuit of happiness." And they rightly did not define happiness. I suggest to you they meant *individual happiness, whatever happiness is to you,* and not a happiness based on a societal norm.

Whatever the reasons, and there are many others than the one just proposed, we begin to not like ourselves, not value ourselves, and feel we're not good enough because we cannot be like everyone else. We find ourselves unable to push our own personal, beautiful, unique shape into the square hole (or whole) of society. Liking ourselves and loving ourselves for who and what we are is paramount to Living In Vibrancy and living the life we desire and ought to be living. And this life is **not** the one we're told we should be living.

We're not supposed to be like anyone else! Let's repeat that. We're not supposed to be like anyone else! Say it out loud right now. **"I'm not supposed to be like anyone else. I'm supposed to be like me."** We are only supposed to be like ourselves. We're supposed to be like ourselves, whatever and whoever that self is. And, just as importantly, we're supposed to like and love ourselves. We have to love ourselves, whoever that self happens to be. And there should not be any judgment of that self.

Native traditions address this idea very succinctly. They are intimate with nature, and so their metaphors and myths are universal ones of nature. Anyone who regularly spends time with nature will understand this completely. If you don't, the next exercise will help you understand the idea of being intimate with nature and alter the metaphors with which you engage the world.

Trees are majestic. Each one is unique in its own beauty and its expression of *treeness*. Yet within and underlying their uniqueness they are all the same. They know their place. They know that they can never, within their lives as trees, be anything more than a tree, solidly rooted in one place for their whole lives, sentry like, watching the cycles of the sun and the seasons, and responding appropriately for their nature. They know exactly what and who they are, and their place in the grand scheme of things. And most importantly, they are radiant in their expression of themselves, always the same, always unique. We don't know what they know. We do not know our place within the grand scheme of things, and we constantly get trapped in being what we're told we're supposed to be instead of being what we know we are.

Experience 1

Work with the energy of a tree. By this I mean first give yourself permission to do something you've never done before, and will probably be told is a strange thing to do. Set aside a couple of hours when you won't be disturbed and have not put any pressures on yourself to be doing anything else. Go to a park or woods and just walk. Walk slowly and enjoy being part of something which is part of you. Walk casually, not focusing on anything in particular, until you find a tree that pulls you. One that you seem naturally drawn towards. One that calls to you personally. This call may come in the form of a voice, or intuition, or inner knowing, or a feeling. They are all valid and the important thing is to honor yourself and your experience.

Walk up to the tree and ask its permission to join it. That's right, ask the tree if it's all right for you to sit with it. Project the question silently with your intent, or come right out and say it out loud. The most important thing is to have your heart open. Whether you speak out loud or silently, project the energy of your question from your heart. Once you feel and intuit an affirmative response, sit down at the tree's base with your back towards it and lean against its trunk. Get comfortable and close your eyes. Let your breathing become slow, easy and rhythmic. As you sit with the tree feel yourself melting into it. Feel your back becoming a trunk with energy coursing from the ground to your tallest limbs. Feel what it's like to be rooted in the earth and to be part of your source and your origin. Understand and experience how it feels to be moved by the wind, to change temperature with the air, and to taste the sun with your leaves. Most importantly feel what it's like to love yourself. Feel with the totality of yourself what it is like to love yourself without pretenses, conditioning, or preconceived ideas for exactly who and what you are. Feel what it's like to love yourself unconditionally for your own magnificent, radiant, unique beauty.

When you feel you're finished, thank the tree. Words are great, but be certain that they come from your heart so that the emotional energy is transferred. The energy is most important. Give the tree a hug. Give yourself one as well. If we don't hug ourselves, how can we expect anyone else to?

Experience 2

Another way to help eliminate the *I'm not good enough* syndrome is to work with a partner and see yourself through their eyes. To do this exercise you need a friend or companion who you feel is in balance and in sync with their life. They don't necessarily have to think they are, but you have to think they are. The person should be someone who you believe in, and who is open to self-exploration and growth. They should be someone who you are able to be open and honest with.

Sit with your partner in a quiet place where you won't be disturbed. You should sit across from each other so you can look into each other's eyes. Have pencils and paper for each of you. Ask your partner to tell you about you. Ask them to list your attributes and assets, and those things they admire about you. You should both consciously open yourself up to the experience. Look into each other's eyes as you are working through this exercise and see *through* your eyes, not *with* them.

Your partner can write down their observations and then share them with you, or speak them as they come into their mind. Initially stick with things you would consider positives. We'll get into negatives later. Gaze into their eyes as they are speaking. Melt into them and see yourself through them. You'll be surprised at the beauty, strength, and power you possess. You will be amazed at the talents and assets you never thought you had. See yourself through the eyes of another and realize that the filters you usually see yourself through are just that, filters which are clouded with the prejudices and insecurities you've been given. See how things you may have thought were bad or negative are in reality assets. Then reverse the process. Give your partner the same gift of perception they have given you.

Next, move on to what we usually think of as negatives. However, we're not going to refer to them as negatives. They are merely personas and energies we need to work with because they no longer serve us. These parts which we consider negative or bad are really assets and attributes which we have outgrown. They have gotten us to where we are now and without them we wouldn't be who we are; but now they are stumbling blocks which hinder us from expressing our own unique beauty. We all have these, every single one of us, and they are not bad. They are our teachers and are with us to guide us into those places we need to travel.

This part calls for surrendering judgment and placing ego aside. Accept what your partner tells you, not as criticisms, but as honest observations. Accept them in love in the same way you accepted the *good* attributes and assets, and understand that they are not negatives, but only observations of things you may or may not want to change. What we call negatives can be turned into some of our greatest gifts and attributes. Fear of death can be turned into a great ally as a hospice volunteer. Excessive worry can transform into the gift of sight and compassion. Shyness can become the most important attribute of an engaging and persuasive orator because that shyness and humbleness speaks to those same parts in every member of an audience.

Everything we have is a gift, and it's up to us to embrace all of them, every single part of ourselves, and use them to the fullest. It's up to us to be authentic to who we are and who we want to be. It's our choice.

If I were her (or him)

We all have historic figures who we admire. These are people who have made some contribution to the history of our world which we believe is significant. Find out who you admire. Who you believe was, or is, great, and worthy of recognition. It doesn't matter if others feel their contribution was significant or worthwhile. All that matters is that you believe in your heart that they did something of value. This person can be someone who did something akin to where your power lies, or they can be someone who has done something not related to anything you have done or ever would want to do. All that matters is that in your estimation they gave our world an incredible gift. For me examples of people like this are Joseph Campbell, and Black Elk, the native North American visionary.

Experience

Find this person who you truly admire and research them. Read everything that's ever been written by them or about them. Learn as much as you can about them and their life. Answer questions about them. Where were they born? To who? What were their circumstances? What perceived obstacles were in their way? Most importantly, what excuses could they have made for letting their power slip by?

Consider contacting the person if they are alive. Open a dialogue. Ask them about their excuses. Ask how they eliminated them. You'll be surprised by the answers. Everyone who has ever done anything had obstacles. And they all had excuses which could have prevented them from doing what they did. And they all eliminated their excuses. Through learning the life story of someone you admire, you will see that they are no different from anyone else, including you. They had the same fears, concerns, and worries. Only they chose to put the excuses aside and be in their power. Being in our power is right for everyone. It's a choice we all can make.

Death

There are no excuses

One of our greatest fears, if not the greatest, is the fear of death. Death is personified as the Grim Reaper. It is portrayed as a vast, forbidding, terrifying unknown–the end of everything–that's going to swallow us up for all of eternity. We're frequently told if we haven't lived a good life, upon our death we are going to sit in front of a harsh, judgmental, punitive deity who has the power to send us to a place of eternal torture and damnation. Death is something to be avoided at all costs, feared, though not really respected, and purposefully pushed out of our consciousness. What's really ironic is that most of our religions believe in an after-life, salvation, and supreme forgiveness, yet we still fear death and passionately avoid any discussion of our own mortality.

Where these ideas and beliefs which cause us to fear death so vehemently originated, and how they became such a huge part of our collective unconscious is not an issue we are going to address. Suffice it to say that like everything else in our life we've been given our perception of death. Our purpose here is to embrace an alternate perception of death, and transform death from a feared enemy into one of our greatest allies and teachers.

The indigenous embrace a perception of death which is completely different than ours. For most native peoples death is a return to our natural, true state of being. Native peoples consider themselves spirits first, spiritual beings having a physical experience, whereas we tend to think of ourselves, our essence, as being physical, that we transform into spirit at death, and that spirit is something we have never been before. For the indigenous our physical lives are merely a pit stop, a way station on the infinite journey of our souls. A native man at the Day of the Dead celebration in Mexico was asked about ghosts. He responded casually to the interviewer, "Senior, we are the ghosts."

For the shaman, the medicine person of native cultures, death is not an enemy to be feared, but a grand and enlightened teacher and ally. A common theme weaving through the medicine traditions of native cultures is the initiation of the shaman through death. Some type of illness or crisis always precedes the shaman's introduction to the world of spirits. This initiation usually takes the form of a spiritual journey or soul flight where the initiate is guided by spirits to the realm of the dead. On this journey, the shaman initiate is introduced to his personal death. He or she dies. There is a true death of the body, the ego, and everything that we usually define as ourselves. Many times this death takes the form of a dismemberment–the initiate sees his or her body being taken apart then put back together. There is a death, and a rebirth, and in the reassembly of the body the person is somehow changed. They now have the ability to communicate with the spirit world. The initiate has faced death, died, and gone beyond the veil of death (our idea of mortality). He or she then returns to the world of matter and time, free in a very real sense. The shaman has faced and stepped past death, and in having done so, has released the stranglehold and claim death has on him. By having died already, the shaman is free to be claimed by life.

The South American medicine tradition handed down through the Q'ero, descendants of the Inca, recognizes that we all have a personal death stalking us, and because of our fear of it, and our fear of our own mortality, we are never able to be truly alive. After facing and going beyond death that fear disintegrates. Death no longer carries a claim over us. Once we are free of the shackles with which death binds us, we can truly be claimed by life. Once we have genuinely accepted and recognized our own mortality, all of our other concerns, worries, and self-pity become insignificant. Death, instead of a feared taker of life, becomes a dear friend. By truly realizing our own mortality death is transformed into a giver of life and bestows upon us the gift of the ability to be in the moment. We learn, with death by our side, that the moments we take for granted will, without question, end at some point. Death clearly informs us that our time on this earth is limited. Any excuses we make for not being and doing what we desire pale in its heavy embrace.

The experiences that follow are designed to help relinquish the fear we have of death and to guide us in personifying our own personal death. The exercises invite our individual, personal death into our lives to help us: 1) recognize our physical mortality, 2) relinquish our fear of death, 3) personify our own personal death, and, 4) transform our death from a feared enemy into a dear teacher, friend, and guide.

As a teacher, friend, and guide, death can show us how to live in the moment, eliminate those excuses that prevent us from doing so, and teach us that the moments of our lives, the ones we take for granted, may end at any time. The experiences will also help you to understand that you are a spirit first, and that absolutely nothing ends with death.

Opening A Dialogue

This is a powerful, yet amazingly simply and easy technique which can be used to dialogue with spiritual entities. It allows the entities to communicate with us in a way that we are familiar with, instead of solely relying on feelings and intuitions from which we have all but have detached ourselves. The technique is so effective that more than one person has stopped midway through the exercise the first time they have done it out of sheer amazement.

Experience

Take a piece of paper and draw a line down the middle from top to bottom. On the left side, at the top, write your name. On the right side, at the top, write Death. Take your pen or pencil, and on the left open a dialogue. Introduce yourself. Begin with, "Hello." Or, "I'm...", or, "My name is..., it's nice to meet you." Next, put your pencil or pen on the right and let death answer through you. Allow the being, in this case the entity we know as death, to answer you through you. Don't be concerned with the nature of the response as it's being written. Just allow it to come. And it will. This is an extremely powerful technique, and the ease with which you get a response may frighten you. These beings we dialogue with are real! And they have things to teach us if we are willing to speak with them, and listen.

Once the response is finished, reply. Put the pen back on the left and write your response. Let the dialogue continue, just as if you are speaking with a friend. Ask your death its name–how should you address it? What does it have to tell you? What excuses does it see you making? How can you eliminate them? When does your death plan to take you? How? How can you change it? Can you renegotiate the deal? Ask your death anything you want. No matter how much we ignore death in our life, it's a certainty, a dead certainty, that we will meet it at some point. By befriending death earlier, rather than later, we can embrace it and have it be an important friend, teacher, and guide within the cycle of our lives.

Your Eulogy

Do you ever wonder how you will be remembered after you've died? Most of us have, at some point in our lives, perhaps when sitting quietly before going to sleep, or in the midst of some crisis or peak moment, or when we were young and starry-eyed and ready to change the world, wondered what people will say about us after we're gone and they think we can't hear them. Will we be remembered for the good we've done? Will people talk about our faults and failures? Who will show up to mourn for us? These are important questions because they reflect on the value of the life we've lived, and on the choices we've made.

Experience

Write your eulogy. Put today's date on the top of your piece of paper and write your eulogy. You've just died. Your death came suddenly and is a tragic loss! How will you be remembered? This is not an obituary: So and so died on Monday, 1999, at 9 a.m. of a heart attack and was survived by.... No. Your eulogy is what will be said about you at your funeral. It's how you will be remembered. Write it. Make it at least one page, but otherwise as long or short as you want. Don't think about it too much, just write it down.

Once you're done, read it. Read your eulogy out loud. Or even better, have someone read it to you. Invite someone close to you to share it with you. Lie down. Cover yourself up. Completely cover yourself from head to toe with a blanket. Listen, as if you are dead, to your eulogy. Is it how you want to be remembered? If so, will you be remembered like that? Reflect on your life and see if how you *want* to be remembered fits with how you *will* be remembered. If they don't fit, what do you need to change in your life so that they do fit?

If what's being said about you is not how you would like to be remembered, how can you change it? What do you need to change in your life so that you will be remembered the way that you want to be remembered? What do you need to do so that when your eulogy is written and read for the last time, it will be exactly what you want to hear?

Lie under the blanket and don't just listen to the words, hear them. Use your kinesthetic sense and hear them with your body. After you've died, will you have lived the life you wanted? Will you be remembered for who you wanted to be? Why did you allow so many excuses to stop you? Eliminate the excuses. Death is waiting!

One Year to Live

You have one year to live. You've just received word and there is no mistake—one year from today's date, at 9p.m. in whatever time zone you are living, the inevitable is going to take place, you are going to die. There is no longer any room for negotiations, promises, or second chances. You will die one year from this moment. You have only one year to live. Now live it.

There have been a number of books written on this specific method of dialoguing with death, and I refer you to them for a more in-depth study. We are all concerned about loss, but when you are dying (as we all in truth are, life is terminal) with the days surely numbered, there really isn't much left to lose. Nothing actually.

Experience

Plan your death. Really plan your last year of life, and death in detail. Who will you have with you when you pass on? What will you say to them? What will your eulogy be? (Glad we did the last exercise? You didn't think you were going to have to use it so soon, did you?) Who will read the eulogy? When will you be buried? Will your body be cremated? Do you want it embalmed? You are dying one year from today. Get a wall calendar and mark the day. Number the days backwards so you can count them down. Make a list of things you would like to do. Is there enough time left?

You will die one year from today. How do those excuses look now? This is real. Your death is imminent. Eliminate the excuses and make your choices now. There's no time left.

A Journey with Death

Death is real, and we need to treat her as such. As we have discussed through much of this book, many of us live in an inanimate world, a place without consciousness, where we have removed all of the spirit. We've created a world and a universe which are very different than ourselves, and we have difficulty relating to things that are different than us.

The indigenous live in an animate, spirit filled, conscious and aware world. Because their world is conscious just as they are, their relationship to it is much different than ours is to our world, and they have little of the difficulty we have relating to the world, because it isn't so alien of a place to them. We don't accept that anything other than people are conscious and aware, yet we have an internal knowing that everything in the world is filled with spirit. We've all had an old car that we've spoken to before we turned the key so that it would start. Likewise, who works with computers who hasn't pleaded with the machine before pushing the print button so that everything comes out right the first time? (I've been talking to mine all morning.) We don't necessarily think of our companion dogs or cats, or any animals for that matter, as conscious in the same sense that we are. But think about your pet. How do you relate to him or her? How do you speak to them? How do you treat her? Probably in a very animate, conscious way, very similar to how you would speak to another person. We generally don't consider trees as aware and conscious, but as you experienced earlier, they are. Trees have a different consciousness and awareness than we're used to, but it's a consciousness and awareness nevertheless. It's the same for all creation. All of creation is conscious, and death is no different. Death was created just like everything else.

This exercise calls for meeting death personally. It calls for putting a face on death and holding hands and walking with him. Now, many of the faces death is going to take are going to be fearful. These images arise from our own ingrained fears which have been heaped upon us since birth. We come into this world with no fears, and certainly no fear of death. We have no idea what death is when we're born, how can we be afraid of it? And because these images are related to fears which we can release, the images can change too. They can transform from gruesome specters to beautiful apparitions.

I recently worked with a client who had been stalked by a fiery demon since she was a child. We met this demon on a journey of healing we took together. Coming face to face with this scarlet devil, I told my client to ask the demon to change into a form that she could recognize, one she could relate to easier, and which didn't hold as much dread for her. She asked it to change, and it did. The demon transformed into a gargoyle. This was better, but still not a form she could relate to without fear. We asked the demon to change again. This time it transformed into a Rottweiler. This was better still, but we still had some work to do. She again asked it to change. This time it became a man, a shadowy, hooded figure with his arms crossed and a sarcastic but playful grin on his face. In this final image she was lying prostrate, tied down by strings which extended from the man's hands. The fiery demon was finally in a form she could engage without fear.

She asked him to release the strings. He said he couldn't. She asked him why? He said he was told by others to keep the strings around her, and that if he released them he would get in trouble. I instructed her to tell him, strongly, without any doubt, to release the strings. She did. He shrugged his shoulders, agreed, and the strings vanished. He also melted away as she floated upwards and experienced a freedom and lightness she had never felt before.

The point of the story is that we create our own demons. There are no devils except those we produce, and we can rid ourselves of them just as easily as we've created them. The same is true of death. Death can be a gruesome demon, as we're used to seeing in the movies, or death can be a kind and gentle friend. It's up to us to choose.

Experience

This experience is done in the same manner as the experiences before when we journeyed. The preparation is the same. A quiet place. No interruptions. Meditation sounds–music, drumming, whatever pleases you. Set your intent, and your focus, to meet death. Verbally ask him or her to come to you. Ask her to be a part of you and make herself known to you. Open yourself up to the experience and let death enter your life.

See what form death takes for you. Is he a black demon or a magenta butterfly? A friend or a foe? Beauty without bound or ugliness incarnate? The death you meet is conscious, whatever form she takes. He is as aware as the tree you've worked with, your companion dog or cat, your spouse, or the last person you spoke to on the phone. Death is conscious and real. If death isn't real, why do we fear him so much?

Whatever form death takes for you, embrace it. Look directly at it. If it's not a form you are comfortable with, tell it to change. Say something like, "Death, change to a form that I can relate to, a form that I won't fear." Don't ask it to take a particular form. For instance, don't say, "Death, become a rose." We can do that sort of thing, but it's not for this exercise. Once you've asked, the form will change. If you don't like the form it becomes, ask death to change again. Keep asking her to change until she has transformed into a form you are comfortable with. It doesn't necessarily have to be a human form, though it certainly can be. Let death be a face, or a cloud, a whisp of smoke, a hooded figure or a skeleton. Whatever form death takes which works for you is appropriate.

Once death is in a form you can relate to, dialogue with it. Ask death about itself. What's it like to be death? Why do we fear it so passionately? What's it like to be so feared? Is it lonely? What lessons does it have for us? What contracts have you made with it? What death have you chosen for yourself? How can you change these deals and contracts if you don't like them? Ask death to show you those things you need to see. Ask your death to advise you, to come into your life and be your companion, friend, and teacher. Ask death about excuses, and the brevity of time. The knowledge that she has for us is indescribable.

We spoke earlier about our fear of death, and said that when we're born we don't have any fear of death. We don't know death so how can we fear it? Ask death to guide you to the place before you were born, before you were ever introduced to her. What's it like to not know death? Did you know her in another form, one that you didn't fear? Was it a form that you accepted as change, not as an end, as light instead of dark? Ask death to take you to her home, the land of the dead. What's it like? Who's there? Talk to them.

Ask death his name. What should you call her? Get personal. She's with you for life. For life, and death.

No Back Doors

We always allow ourselves back doors, and back doors are intimately related to our excuses. A back door is a way out, a fall back. It's a cushion we can use if things don't work out the way we want. We're taught that we need these back doors for security. The problem with back doors is they stop us from being one hundred percent committed to what we are doing. A back door breaks the unbending intent and focus of attention we need to choose and create the world we desire.

Back doors come in many forms. They usually have an *if* attached to them. I can get divorced *if* the marriage doesn't work. *If* my business doesn't succeed, I can go back to doing whatever I did before. *If* I can't finish the workout, I can just go and take a steam. *If* it doesn't work, I can just.... You finish the sentence. We drown ourselves in negative *ifs* and the false security these *ifs* give us.

Back doors are about the old saying cautioning us about putting all of our eggs in one basket. "Don't put all of your eggs in one basket," we're told. "*What if...?*" Yet if we don't put all of our eggs in the one basket, the basket will never be full. And when we're not committed one hundred percent to who and what we want to be, our lives aren't full either. Back doors are an excuse, one of the biggest, and we need to eliminate them. Once we eliminate the back doors, front doors we cannot imagine open up for us.

Experience

Remember back to a situation in your life that was completely untenable. One that was just unbearable and you saw no way out. A situation where there was no back door you could find, anywhere. A situation where you had no choice but to go forward. How did it turn out? It probably turned out just fine. Probably even better than fine, and certainly better than you ever imagined it would turn out. Make a list of all of these situations which have been part of your life. There have been many where you have chosen the front door, even if only by default because there was no back door. How have these turned out? Much better than you could have imagined.

Think of a situation where you chose the back door. There probably have been many. What happened when you chose the back door? You probably went back to your same usual life, the life you are trying to step away from. Imagine if you had chosen the front door. What possibilities may have opened up for you if you had gone forward instead of backwards?

Next, put yourself in a situation where you don't have any of the usual back doors. You can pick any situation you like, but for this experience let's use the following scenario. You're in a foreign city. You've been left stranded. You don't have any money, not a penny, and you don't have any place to stay. You don't have contacts, you don't speak the language, and you only have the clothes on your back. What do you do? You need to survive. If you make excuses about doing things you're not comfortable with, you'll die. You can't afford to have any back doors. In fact, there aren't any.

Where does this scenario take you? What options open up for you? See how resourceful you are when you need to be. See how powerful and inventive you are when you need to be. Sit with the situation and allow the possibilities to open up for you.

Take it a step further. Make it real. Have someone drop you in a strange town. You have no money and no identification. Nothing. Make a plan that they will be back to pick you up in a few days at a predetermined place. But you need to survive until then. There are no excuses for you because there cannot be–this is real.

Excuses are one of the biggest stumbling blocks we face on our journeys towards who we want to be. Yet all of the excuses we use are only valid because we allow them to be valid. We've been handed them, and accepted them without protest as truths in our lives.

Eliminate your excuses and feel what it's like to be alive without any excuses for being who you can be. Feel what it's like to be someone you always thought you couldn't be. Eliminate the excuses, close the back doors, and step into who you want to be! It's simply a matter of choice. And it's your choice. Choose!

FOUR

Step Into
The Empty Space

He does not see, does not apprehend, for that which transcends all categories cannot be apprehended.

Henry Corbin

THE EMPTY SPACE is known by many names–the Void, the place of being/non-being, source, God, the timeless, the eternal now. We have put many labels on this concept because none of them are truly appropriate, because the concept transcends categories and cannot be apprehended by our normal consciousness. We call it the Void, but it's not really void of anything–it's completely filled with potential. Everything that has ever happened, can happen, and will happen arises from it. It's the place of potential, the realm of creation, and the space of pure, unadulterated consciousness and knowing. And the importance of the Empty Space cannot be overstated. It's where the incessant chatter of our minds, which upholds the world we've been given, stops. It's where the who we've been told we are melts away, and where our true self mingles and melts with our creative potential. It's where we step past all judgment of right and wrong and become all that is. It's where we create our reality from. First, we will learn to Step into the Empty Space, then we will learn to create from within it by Choosing Our Circle.

The Empty Space is a realm we've all visited, although we don't realize it. When we are in the Empty Space, the world as we know it stops, and we live in the universe of imagination and dreams. These worlds are as real as ours, we have just not been taught to honor and accept them. Yet everything that exists in our world, everything we have created from faxes to pagers, from candles to rockets, existed in the imaginal realm until it was brought from there to here by someone who caused it to become manifest in time and space. We all have the innate ability to visit the Void, it's our Source. And we all have the ability to bring gifts, including the life we desire, from the realm of the imaginal to our world of time and space. All we have to do to comprehend this truth is look around.

Getting to the Empty Space is easy. We all have some activity that takes us to a place where time ceases to flow, the world stops, and we are communing with the activity, ourselves, our world and the whole of creation. It is in this Empty Space where we meet God, and the God we meet is merely a reflection of what is within each of us.

A year ago I worked with a couple having marital difficulties. We worked from the standpoint of perception and used shamanic techniques so they could see each other with different eyes–each other's. One of the difficulties they had was arguing over who was going to mow the lawn. They each would rush to beat the other to the activity. It was the most mowed lawn in town. Mowing the lawn for each of them was their connection to the Empty Space. Within the activity of mowing the lawn they each found a place where time stopped, they were at peace, and creation entered their world. I refer to mowing the lawn as an activity because it wasn't a job or a task for either of them, it was a meditation, and an act of love and creation.

The woman talked about how when she was mowing the lawn seemed to guide her. She would make circles and ellipses, patterns of all types. Her own crop circles I guess. In performing this seemingly mundane task the world as she knew it stopped, and she existed wherever, whenever, and as whoever she chose.

Running is one of my avenues to the Empty Space. I'm no marathoner. I enjoy a nice, slow, leisurely jog. When I'm running, time stops, my mind as I'm used to it working stops, and ideas and thoughts from the imaginal realm flow freely. It's where the majority of my ideas for stories and workshops come from. Ideally, our connection to the place of timelessness is what we do for the majority of our lives–our work. For most of us, however, this is unfortunately not the case.

My father was a house painter for the majority of his life–over 30 years. It's hard work. I know. I worked with him summers and weekends when I was growing up. And he always worked 6 or 7 day weeks. I never understood that. I knew it wasn't for the money. And it wasn't to just, "get out of the house." He and my mother had a good relationship. I could never understand why he worked so hard. Neither could I understand why it never seemed like work to him. It certainly was to me. It was hard work to me.

Yet for him, it was just what he did. Finally, one summer, I understood my father.

My father was at my house painting a sun room that had just been remodeled. It was midmorning and I was upstairs writing. I went to the kitchen to get a cup of coffee and then to see if he needed anything. I stepped into the doorway leading to the room he was painting. His back was towards me. He was painting the windows–the wooden frames around the glass. I stood there in silence watching him as the brush in his hand glided effortlessly back and forth tenderly burnishing the glossy white paint over the wood. There was an indescribable energy in that room. It held a feeling of passion, a love in a sense that we are wholly unfamiliar with. My father was present, yet he wasn't. He was in the room physically, but his presence was elsewhere.

As I gazed at the slightly overweight man with graying black hair hardly covering the skin at the top of his head, I understood. I understood all of those things that I never had all of those years when I got up at 6 a.m. to go to work with him. He wasn't working in the sense that we're used to the word. He was in the timeless. He was basking and effortlessly floating in the realm of spirit where there is nothing but beauty, wholeness, and love. He was in the Empty Space and eternity was embracing him. He had spent his life there.

After watching him for a minute and soaking up as much of the energy and beauty of the moment as I could, I cleared my throat and asked him if he wanted some coffee. Without pausing he answered, "Yeah. Sure, Rick." He nodded his head to the left, brush never hesitating. "My cup's over there," he said. I walked in, picked up the cup and walked out. He never left the Empty Space. It's part of him. And he's part of it. Thank you Dad. I love you.

To this day, I don't believe that he understands the concept of the Empty Space. At least as far as the intellectualizations we're making within this book in order to try to do something we never will, and that is, understand the Empty Space. But that doesn't matter. And it doesn't matter if he ever understands. My father has something more important than understanding. He has experience. He has the experience of the Empty Space. He has knowledge. He has lived it.

In the shamanic traditions, we make a distinction between information and knowledge. One of my teachers uses the example that information is knowing the chemical composition of water–H_2O. Knowledge is knowing how to make it rain. Likewise, in the medicine traditions we say that change happens instantaneously, but that understanding comes later, or may never come. The understanding is not what's important. What is important is the knowledge. And this knowledge only comes through experience, or direct contact with Source, not from intellectualizations.

We don't have to understand the Empty Space or the transcendent. In fact, we can't and never will, and that information is hard for our rational self to accept. The intellectualizations we make are only to satisfy our left brained, rational side; but there comes a time when we have to tell that part of ourselves, "Thanks, but no thank you. I appreciate your help, but I don't need you right now." We don't need to understand the Empty Space, we need to feel it. We need to experience and live it. That's why this book is titled, *Living The Steps to Vibrancy*, not *Understanding The Steps To Vibrancy*. Now, let's Step into the Empty Space.

We are going to begin with exercises that use activities we're familiar with, things which have taken us to the Empty Space already, though we didn't know we were there. Once we're somewhat familiar with the territory, we will step into more traditional meditations and use art and poetry to produce an aesthetic arrest, a stopping of the functioning of our minds which uphold the world we know. Relinquishing our minds puts us into the place between thoughts, the place where creation occurs. Once there, we can assume our true nature, and create.

What Do I Do?

What do you do that takes you to the Empty Space? What activity is there that propels you into a place of timelessness? A place where you aren't aware of the world around you. A place where a whole day just disappears. A place where you feel whole, complete, and fulfilled. Every one of us has an activity which takes us to this place, the Empty Space. We all do. It's only a matter of remembering and realizing. I have a dear friend who is a sound engineer. He can spend hours upon hours working and reworking recordings until they are just right. It's one of his avenues to the Empty Space. Have you ever watched people fishing? People who like to fish step into the Empty Space as soon as they cast the line. For most of us, tirelessly waiting for a fish to bite is an unimaginable boredom. The fisher is residing in the Empty Space where their spirit is soaring and dancing in imaginal realms as real as the rod and reel, line, hook, and fish.

Experience

Sit down, relax, go into your private, sacred place, and remember your avenue, your on-ramp to the Empty Space. It may be an activity in your life now. It may not be a part of your life now. It may be something you did when you were younger that you, "just don't have the time for anymore." Relax and casually focus on your breaths. Let your breaths become rhythmic and flowing, set your intent to remember your path to the Empty Space, and allow your mind to float. Allow the thoughts and images to drift in and out of your consciousness and remember what your link to the Empty Space is. What is it that you used to do, or do now, that makes time stop? What activity makes you feel whole? What activity makes the world as you know it disappear? Use your kinesthetic sense. What is it that makes your body feel at ease and relaxed, and in perfect, absolute harmony and balance?

Once you know what the activity is, and it can be as mundane as changing the cat litter, watering the roses, or vacuuming, it doesn't matter, bring yourself into it. Remember the activity, not only with your mind but with your whole body and your whole being. Recall what it's like to be doing the activity which makes time stop for you. Go within and feel yourself doing whatever the activity is. Engage in the activity at a visceral level and become aware of how your body feels. What are your thoughts? Where is your mind? Where are you? While you're engaged in the activity, feel what the Empty Space is like. You're in it. Don't become trapped by trying to understand it, you won't. Become cognizant of it. Become aware of the Empty Space through feeling and intuition. Don't attempt to use words to describe and remember it, the Empty Space lies beyond categorizations, but acknowledge it through bodily sensation and experiential knowledge. Learn its territory through your experience of it and let that experience become your map. It's the place of creation. The place where your self and your mind as you know them stops. Judgments, prejudices, and old contracts melt away and you—the *real self*—enters the imaginal realm of creation and potential. It's where you create the reality and the life of your choice.

Next, give yourself the gift of the time to do it. Whatever the activity is, bring it into your life. Do whatever it is that takes you to the Empty Space, the place of timelessness and creation. Allow yourself the freedom to engage in it daily, if even for only 30 minutes. That half hour will do more for getting you to where you would like to be than days of struggle. We tend to think of these kinds of activities as *time outs*. We view them as time outs from the real world, and that they have no real value other than to relax us so that we can reenter the rat race filled with energy. They are time outs. They are time outs from the world we have been handed so that we can create the world we desire. Time out is not time lost, although we are used to thinking it is. It's within these time outs that the real work is done. Where do you think our world comes from? It's in the time outs that creation occurs. The time ins are when we allow the creation to manifest in our lives and our world.

In the shamanic traditions the first thing the shaman does in the morning is take a time out and step into the Empty Space. In the Empty Space, the medicine person assembles their day. The shamans believe that if you don't assemble your own day, then you have to settle for the day someone else assembles for you. Most of us wander through our lives living the days other people all too readily assemble for us.

Take a moment each morning to assemble your day. *Be* in the Empty Space–It's home.

Will I See The Sun Tomorrow?

The Empty Space is the timeless. And this is literal. There is no time in the Empty Space. There is no past or future. Everything is in the present. Everything that has ever happened, will happen, and can happen is present and available in a timeless moment of now.

Now the logical reaction to a statement like this is, "That's impossible. There has to be a past and a future."

Why? Our experience of linear time, of past, present, and future is all that we know. It's the way the physical world we're part of, by virtue of our physical bodies, works. Because we only have this one experience, we tend to believe it's the only way it can be. If you order a particular food in a restaurant that you've never had before and it's badly prepared, you may never order it again. You may never order it again because you have had that one experience and you believe it will always be like that. It's all you know based on your experience. It may be that the dish is something you would enjoy beyond belief if it is properly prepared, but your whole world of that particular food is that it tastes like it did the one time you ate it. There is no other way. Years ago I ordered swordfish in a restaurant. It was badly prepared, although I didn't know it at the time because I had never had it before. I got very sick and it wasn't until years later that I ordered it again. My experience was different. My perception of it changed, and it's now one of my favorite foods.

Our concept of time is like this. Even though modern physics has proven intellectually that time is variable and malleable, we don't experience it as such. We don't believe that it's possible for there to be a time where there is no past, present, or future because we've never had the experience. The understanding of concepts is nice, but it's the experience of them which brings us in line with true knowledge, and then allows us to utilize this knowledge.

Being in the Empty Space is beauty beyond comprehension. It's poetry. But, as physical beings, we exist in a world of time and space. To bring the Empty Space into our lives, to bring timelessness into the field of time and space, means living in the present. It means making every moment *now*, and, *being* totally in the moment. I don't really like the use of the phrases, "living in the present," or "being in the present." The word "present," because of the glasses of perception we've been given, is usually associated with past and future. Saying present for most of us immediately connects us to past and future. While we have no perfect word to describe something indescribable, "now" is a better choice. Now means now. Now, not later. There is only the *now*, and nothing else. Being in the now means being only in the moment, the moment of now, and this is the timeless, the Empty Space within the field of time and space.

Experience 1

The eternal now has been approached in many different ways by the various spiritual traditions, and we can approach this idea of being in the eternal now from many different angles. First, write down all of the thoughts you've had so far today. If you're reading this in the morning, you've got it made. If it's night and you've had a long day, it's going to be a little tougher. Without thinking about it, write down all of the things you've thought about during the course of the day. Everything, or at least as many of the thoughts as you can think of. Now look at the list. Put a "P" next to the thoughts you had about events which occurred in the past. Put a "F" next to the thoughts you've had about the future. Put a "N" next to thoughts which had to do with things which were happening in the present for you when you had the thought about them. Add up all of the P's, F's, and N's, and compare the numbers.

We spend the majority of our lives either reliving or haunted by a past which is just that, past, and worrying about a future that we have no guarantee will ever come. We spend very little time truly being in the moment, being in the now, yet the now is where we always are, and it's where we create from. The present moment is a gift, that's why it's called the present. Each moment is a gift, one that may cease arriving at any moment.

Experience 2

Our new friend Death can help us to be fully in the present. Death can come and snatch us out of the field of time and space any time. Any time. Just turn on the news and you'll see this is true. There is absolutely no guarantee that you will live to finish reading this book. And that's true even if you plan on speed reading and finishing it within the next couple of hours. Odds are in your favor that you will, but we'll see in the next chapter that odds really don't matter. There is absolutely no certainty that you will live to finish reading this book. None whatsoever. And there is no certainty that you will see the sun tomorrow. Absolutely none. There is no one hundred percent money back guarantee.

Invite Death, you're now on an intimate basis with her–you know each other by name–to come and sit with you. Meditate or journey with Death and ask her to help you embody the notion that there really is no guarantee that you will see the sun rise tomorrow. Let him help you to understand at a visceral, cellular level that there is not even a guarantee you will be able to finish the meditation without him beckoning you with a crooked finger and saying, "Come on now, it's time to come with me for good." Ask Death to let you *feel and know* the fact–The Fact–that he can take you any time. Through death know, feel, and experience your own physical mortality. Ask Death to show you how to be in the now all of the time. Ask Death to show you how to be in the moment, because the next moment may not come. Today's sunrise may have been your last.

Only Words?

Words and affirmations are powerful tools for coalescing thoughts and manifesting the imaginal into our ordinary, physical reality. Words are a first step in transforming thoughts into physical reality, and this knowledge has been echoed throughout history from the Buddha who said, "We are what we think we are," to John Locke's famous statement, "I am who I remember I am," to the more contemporary Kurt Vonnegut Jr. who commented that, "We have to be careful what we think (and say) we are, because we'll become it." And the most powerful words of all, "I am..." You finish the sentence.

In the Oriental Reiki system of healing being in the now is of critical importance. We will borrow its affirmations as a way of stepping out of the past, present, and future, and into the now. In Reiki practice everyday is seen as new. Each day is seen as new potential, a new beginning, a new creation, and a new gift. The Reiki affirmations focus our attention to that singular moment that we call a day, one, and only one day at a time. As we've experienced, there is no guarantee there will be another day.

The affirmations all begin with, "Just for today...." One version of the Reiki affirmations reads:

> *Just for today I will live the attitude of gratitude.*

> *Just for today I will not worry.*

Just for today I will not anger.

Just for today I will do my work honestly.

*Just for today I will show love and respect
for every living thing.*

The Reiki affirmations go directly to the heart of who we are and who we aspire to be. They truly echo the words of the Buddha, "See yourself in others. Then whom can you hurt? What harm can you do?"

Experience

Write your own set of affirmations. Begin each one with, "Just for today...." Make them meaningful and applicable to your own personal journey. Some suggestions are:

Just for today I will live completely in the moment.

Just for today I will not say, "I can't."

Just for today I will love freely, unconditionally.

Just for today I will do whatever I need to be my best.

Just for today I will be responsible.

Just for today I won't make any excuses.

Just for today I will *be for today*, I won't think about tomorrow.

Use the affirmations for this exercise, and then be creative and use affirmations with any of the exercises in this book. You can use affirmations for whatever you want. Affirmations work, that's why everyone suggests that you use them. But you have to use them. Say them out loud as often as you need in order to keep the ideas and energy they carry with you and to maintain your focus on them. Use your affirmations to keep yourself in the moment. Use them to stay in the *now*. When you are in the now, the past doesn't exist, and the future is whatever you desire it to be.

Thought to Thought

Listen to a fast drum beat. The boom–boom–boom echoes in your ears. Your body resonates with the rhythmic, methodic pulsation. Now listen more carefully. Between each beat, between each thump of the beater against the taut skin is a tiny space of silence. It's minute and not noticed, but it's there. If you don't believe me look at the equalizer bar on the stereo. Between each vibrant pulse of sound the readout drops back to zero. Within the seemingly continuous, unbroken chain of sounds are a series of Empty Spaces. These are true places of silence within the flurry of sounds.

We are no different. Our images of ourselves and our whole world are upheld by our thoughts. We drift from one thought to another in an apparently continuous fashion, each thought following closely on the heels of the prior thought, and each one continually reinforcing the world that we call real. One thought feeds another, which feeds another, which feeds still the next. They have to feed each other in order to persistently uphold the consensual world we're used to.

But these thoughts of ours are not as continuous and unbroken as we believe. Incandescent light filaments flicker on and off 60 times per second, yet they seem to provide a continuous light because we are not normally sensitive enough to see the flicker. It's the same with our thoughts. They flicker on and off so fast that we don't realize they're doing it. Between our thoughts, which uphold the world, is the place where the self we're used to believing is our real self, is not thinking. The question becomes, "Who are you between your thoughts? Who are you when your mind is not upholding an image of itself?"

What is it that lies between our thoughts? The Empty Space. Between our thoughts is the Empty Space, and within this void of timelessness is our personal and collective Source. It's where the true self, the I AM, exists. It's where the self we're used to sources from. It's where the real you which is beyond past, present, and future exists within the eternal now and is available to create anything and everything because it *is* the divine spark of potential and creation within all of us.

Experience

The Empty Space is the space between our thoughts. Find the place, the space between your thoughts. Go to the quiet, sacred area you've created for yourself where you have been doing these exercises. Quiet your breaths. Let them become soft, easy, and rhythmic. Next, become aware of your thoughts. Become aware of your thoughts in their usual state–floating and flowing, apparently ceaseless, one into another. What are your thoughts? Are they thoughts about your breathing? Your meditation? About your job? What's for dinner? When are you going to mow the lawn? Become aware of your thoughts, and instead of trying to push them away, let them flow. Allow your thoughts to just come. Whatever they are, however many there are, accept them. As the thoughts flow, look for the space between them. The space is there. No matter how fast it seems that the thoughts are coming, there is a tiny space between each and every one of them. Set your intent to find that space. You'll get there. You'll step into the space between your thoughts.

At first, you will only step into the space between your thoughts for infinitesimally short periods of time. You may not even remember. But you'll have been there. Then, as you become more familiar with the territory, it will become easier, and the time you spend between your thoughts will be longer.

As the time between your thoughts becomes longer and you perceive the Empty Space more and more, ask yourself: Who is this between my thoughts? Who am I when I'm not thinking? How do I feel when I'm in the Empty Space? In a sense, step back and become an observer of your thoughts instead of the thinker. Who is this observer? You'll be surprised at the answer!

There are many aids you can use to find this place between your thoughts. One aid is a drum beat. As we've discussed, a drum beat is very engaging for most people and rapidly induces a meditative state of consciousness. And, as we have mentioned, we're used to listening to the sound of the beat and not looking for the space between the sounds. Put on a drumming tape as a guide to your meditation. However, instead of listening to the sound of the drum, listen for the space between the sounds. Set your intent and focus your awareness on finding the silence between each beat. This is a powerful technique which will quickly pull you into the Empty Space.

Alternately, if drumming is distracting to you, try a metronome. A metronome is a device we've all seen but might not know its name. It's the device musicians sometimes use to keep a beat. Generally, it is a vertical bar with a weight attached that slides up and down. The bar is set in motion from side to side and it clicks each time it moves through a cycle. Set the metronome at about 60 beats per minute and focus on the sound between the ticks. As you get better at the technique, increase the rate slowly until it's 120 or so beats per minute. Still, keep your focus on the silence between the ticks and allow the silent spaces to guide you into the Empty Space. Using a metronome is a powerful way of accessing the Empty Space.

The Poetry of Life

Poetry is a marvelous and incredibly beautiful vehicle for carrying, and sometimes catapulting us into the Empty Space. It's a perfect vehicle to ride into the timeless, because the Empty Space is where the poetry comes from. Poets spend a good portion of their lives in the Empty Space bringing the gifts it has to offer us back within their words. The Empty Space, the transcendent, is beyond words. It's beyond any description that our languages can afford. And that's the way it's supposed to be. By definition, the transcendent is that which transcends all categories–categories being the logical constructs of our rational minds–so it cannot be apprehended and understood rationally. It's a place of feelings and intuitions. It's a realm of direct experience and passion. Good poetry takes us to a place of feeling and emotion that we cannot directly access with words. Poetry allows us to know, through words, those things we can know—meaning experience—but cannot speak about. Poetry gives us the gift of *experiencing*, not understanding, the incomprehensible.

I recently saw the movie *Contact*. I enjoyed it, but am not going to make this a review. One of the best parts, from the perspective we're working with, was when Jodi Foster was on her voyage into the unknown. One of the reasons she was picked to take the voyage was because she was a scientist and was supposed to be able to understand and document the mysteries she was going to encounter. At one point, she is hanging, literally, on the edge of forever. The images of the filmmaker's dream of creation and eternity were swirling around her. As she floated on the brink of the timeless, trying to describe what she was witnessing, she uttered the line, "They should have sent a poet."

They should have sent a poet! She had no words to describe the majestic beauty and awe inherent in the act of creation she was witnessing and more importantly, experiencing. The Great Mystery is just that, a Great Mystery, and will forever elude us if we remain fixed within our scientific, mechanistic paradigms. Poets, however, can describe the indescribable in a way that we cannot necessarily understand, but that more importantly, we can feel and experience. And as we've seen over and over, it's the *experience*, not the understanding, that truly matters.

Following is a short poem by the 13th Century Sufi poet, Rumi.

> *Late, by myself, in the boat of myself,*
> *no light and no land anywhere,*
> *cloudcover thick. I try to stay*
> *just above the surface, yet I'm already under*
> *and living within the ocean.*

You just cannot know intellectually what these words mean. They don't make sense intellectually and their meaning transcends intellectual thought. Yet you can feel and experience what they mean if you sit quietly with them and allow them to percolate through your body, mind, and spirit right down to the level of your soul.

Experience 1

Buy a book of poetry. It doesn't matter who the poet is. It doesn't really matter what the poem is about. The important thing is you find a poem that speaks to you in a personal manner. If you aren't ready to make the leap and buy a book of poetry, there are poems scattered throughout this book. There are also three magical poems at the end of this chapter.

Meditate with the poem. By that I mean go to your private, sacred space. Read the poem, first with your mind and intellect, then with your heart and the I AM who inhabits the Empty Space. Read the poem out loud, and as you read it, listen to, and hear the words. Intellectualize and try to make rational sense out of the poem. You won't be able to. But in trying, you'll be suspending your thoughts because a paradox which can't be solved by your rational side will be forming. Out of this dissonance you'll reach a place of euphoric disorientation where nothing will seem right, yet you'll be wholly at ease and relaxed. This moment, with rationality and intellect suspended, is the time to feel and experience the poem the way it is meant to be experienced. What do you feel? What emotions are stirred by the poem? Let yourself be carried by the sensations and feelings behind the words. What images arise? Where do they take you? How does it feel to embrace the timeless within the field of time and space? What is your source?

Experience 2

Once you've become familiar with the territory of poetry, write the poem of your life. Our lives are our art, and we all have a *poetry of being* we never touch. Write the poem of your life. Don't worry if it's good enough–there is no such thing as good enough or not good enough. Don't concern yourself with whether or not it will ever be published. It's yours, and whatever you write is beautiful because it is your own unique expression of creation. Write the poem of your life. What is its verse? What is its rhythm? Does it rhyme? What is its Source? Your Source? See your life as a seamless flow, a tidal rhythm that only changes and never ends.

Art

Works of art can also rapidly carry us into the Empty Space. Art has been described as functional and non-functional. An example of functional art is a uniquely designed chair or an unusually styled lamp. These things are pleasing to look at but also have a specific function. Non-functional art is art which has no purpose other than to be viewed, or better said, *seen.* It is something which has no recognizable function. Examples of this type of art might include a sculpture like the Picasso in Chicago, or an abstract painting, or a mobile composed of unrecognizable characters. All art can produce an aesthetic arrest–a stoppage of our minds and thoughts. This aesthetic arrest is similar to the euphoric disorientation we referred to earlier. With functional art we need to look past its use and beyond its functionality in order to get to this point, and that is sometimes difficult to do. A pen or ash tray can produce an aesthetic arrest, but it's very difficult for us to change our perceptions and look past their functionality. Non-functional art on the other hand has no identifiable use. Because we don't have any preconceived or ingrained notions about a piece of non-functional art, it's easier to reach a place of aesthetic arrest through viewing it than by looking at a piece of art which has a function. This aesthetic arrest is then a catapult into the Empty Space.

Experience

Find a piece of art that speaks to you—one to which you feel an uncanny attachment, that you enjoy immensely, and are pulled towards with an almost magnetic force. It can be anything–a painting in a museum, a picture in a magazine, a knickknack you picked up as a gift, anything that you are pulled towards and beckoned by. The only caveat is the art should have absolutely no discernible function. It should absolutely not have any purpose you can think of, and not include any commonly recognizable elements.

Again, it doesn't matter what the piece of art is. It can be a stone you picked up on a walk, a stick, driftwood, or a few colored lines on a piece of paper. The art can be anything, just so you have an attraction to it, and it has no functionality for you.

As before, go to your sacred place. Put the piece of art a comfortable distance in front of you at eye level. (The distance will depend upon the size of the piece of art.) Orient yourself, get comfortable, and gaze at it. Just relax, slow your breathing, be comfortable, and gaze. *Be* with it, and *see* it. Don't try to do anything with it. Don't consciously attempt to make it stop your thoughts. Just sit with it and gaze at it. Give yourself to the art and allow it to carry you into the Empty Space. What does it transform into as you look at it? What feelings well up in you? Where does it take you? Allow the process of aesthetic arrest to take place. Allow the process to stop your normal thinking and put you in a state of euphoric disorientation. Allow yourself to be carried into the Empty Space. Go to the Empty Space, just *be*, and experience the wonder of wholeness.

I'm In The Empty Space Now what?

So, you're in the Empty Space. It feels grand. You're basking in the radiance of the timeless. You know what it's like to experience wholeness, completion, and ecstasy. You've tasted Source, your true self, and the I Am of creation. Now what? How does this help you to Live in Vibrancy? How does this help you to experience the *Glow of Being Alive*?

The Empty Space is where creation occurs. It's where we create from. It's the place where we are not only in touch with the creative source, *we are* the creative source. That's right, within the Empty Space *we are* the Creative Source. Any thoughts we have are mandates to create. A single thought with no other thoughts contradicting it, or opposing it, is creation, and will be manifest. Let me repeat that. A single thought with no other thoughts contradicting it, or opposing it, is creation, and will be manifest. Once we have silenced all of our thoughts any single, pure, unadulterated thought is an act of creation. We can now understand the real importance of The Steps to Vibrancy: All of the thoughts, commands, and ways of thinking we've been given need to be released so that there is nothing, absolutely nothing opposing our creative command.

This principle has been called many names. It's known as will, intent, focus of attention, pure purpose. They're all the same. They all imply a complete, total, unopposed focus of attention. This attention and focus has to be so totally and completely upon a certain thought or idea that it fills the mind and crowds all other ideas out of our consciousness and our unconscious.

The point of getting to the Empty Space is twofold. One, to feel and experience at a visceral level just who and what we truly are. To know the sensations of eternity and wholeness. To feel and experience that we are more than we ever imagined, and that our perceptions of ourselves are severely limited, and limiting. And two, to create. The Empty Space is where creation arises from, and it arises from us. When our minds are clear, empty, and unclouded, and we bring in a pure, unopposed thought, it is a mandate to create. It plants the seed of becoming into the fabric of the Void from where time and space emerge. It's simply up to us to choose what that seed is. Once we've walked through the Circles of Emergence and Chosen Our Circle, we will learn how to plant, nurture, and harvest the fruits of this seed.

Three Poems to
Step Into The Empty Space

If the beloved is everywhere,
The lover is a veil,
But when living itself
Becomes the Friend,
Lovers disappear.

Rumi

Lost

Stand still. The trees ahead and bushes beside you
Are not lost. Wherever you are is called Here.
And you must treat it as a powerful stranger,
Must ask permission to know it and be known.
The forest breathes. Listen. It answers,
I have made this place around you,
If you leave it you may come back again, saying Here.
No two trees are the same to Raven.
No two branches are the same to Wren.
If what a tree or a bush does is lost on you,
You are surely lost. Stand still. The forest knows
Where you are. You must let it find you.

Native American Elder

Brown Leaves

Three men feeding a fire with brown leaves:
two disappear, after a time, return,
while the last stands watch, rolls up his sleeves,

though the air is cold and the earth still heaves
in its sleep. They don't display much concern,
three men feeding a fire with brown leaves,

but then each of them in his heart believes
he will contain the flames, they will not burn
beyond his limit, as a dog who grieves

for a lost litter soon forgets, or cleaves
to some other love, bed or bowl in turn,
three men feeding a fire with brown leaves.

The flies begin to stir beneath the eaves.
Only those who cannot feel it must learn
that fire germinates, that the pod reaves

in the wind, that time alone relieves
the pressure of our promise, or what pattern
three men feeding a fire with brown leaves
will discern, what fabric our knowledge weaves.

Revan Schendler

FIVE

Choose Your Circle

The field is the only reality.
Albert Einstein

AS WE HAVE DISCUSSED, "Reality is those myths we haven't quite seen through yet." In this, one of Joseph Campbell's most repeated thoughts, you can easily substitute paradigm, or belief system, for myth. Reality is those paradigms or beliefs we haven't quite seen through yet. A paradigm is a world view. It is a particular way of organizing the world and our reality. It is a set of beliefs which we use to engage the world. No single paradigm or belief system is more real than another, or better than another. In the Western world our shared, consensual world view is an inanimate, mechanistic paradigm. Our world is ordered upon the assumptions, not facts, that we are the only things truly alive and conscious, we are separate from everything else, and the universe is governed by laws and absolute truths which are independent of us and that we can come to know. Our world is ordered on the premise of a pure subject–object relationship, and that the subject and object do not and cannot affect each other.

The indigenous, as we have seen, have an animate, spirit filled, complementary way of ordering the world. For them *everything* is alive and conscious. People are not separate from anything, but part of and intimately related to *every thing*, including each other. For the indigenous, the laws which govern the universe change as our perception of them changes, and there really is no object, only subject–subject. Neither paradigm is more real, but the reality where we are intimately part of an eternal dance of consciousness and life is infinitely more fulfilling and empowering.

The Circles of Emergence are a set of three paradigms, three ways we can live in, order, and create our world. None is more real than another. They are all real, some are just more familiar to us. Imagine three concentric circles. That is, a large circle containing a smaller circle, and then another still smaller circle within the second.

The First Circle, the smallest and center circle, is Certainty. It's the place where most of us live our lives. It's the place of, "I'm never going to be able to do that, so why even try." Or, "That's just the way it is, I can't change it." The Second Circle, the middle one, is the realm of probabilities, and it's where some people live. It's the place of, "My mother had cancer, so I'll probably have it too. But, maybe not." It's a place of indecision, or rather, a place where we allow the consensual to decide for us. The Second Circle, the realm of probabilities, is a better paradigm, and a more empowering way of existing in and engaging the world, but there is yet a still more empowering alternative.

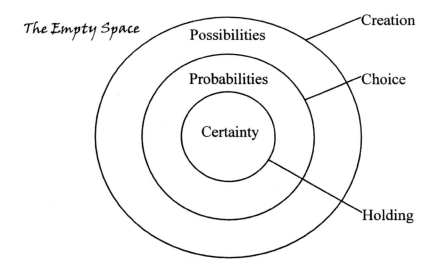

The Circles of Emergence

The interface between the First Circle and the Second Circle is Holding. This is holding onto old ways of thinking that don't serve us. It's holding onto beliefs we've been given but never examined ourselves to see whether or not they're valid, or if they are a choice we've made for the way we want to live in the world.

The Third Circle, the largest and outermost of the three, is the realm of Possibilities. It's the place of, "I can do that, there's no reason I can't. Nothing is impossible." As we'll see, reaching the Third Circle closes a circle. It brings us back to a place of certainty, but here the certainty is the certainty which we choose. It's the certainty we create where odds and the consensual no longer matter. It's the most empowering state of existence, one that's our birthright, but one few people recognize as possible, or choose.

The interface between the Second Circle and Third Circle is Choice. We can choose the way we live. We can choose our paradigms and beliefs systems. We can choose our world and our reality. There is an eternity filled with an infinity of possibilities. The Third Circle says, "Choose one." Someone gave me a bumper sticker that reads, "The universe accommodates itself to my view of reality." That's true, and that is living in the Third Circle.

Beyond the Third Circle is the Void. And we've been there already. It's the Empty Space. It's the place of the mystic, the realm of pure creation. It's the domain of *All Possibilities*. The place of pure existence. The interface between the Empty Space and the Third Circle is Creation. The interface is manifestation of potential, possibilities, and vision in our world, the playing field of time and space. Returning from the Empty Space, from beyond the Third Circle, we bring the vision of our lives into our reality.

Certainty
The First Circle

We live in a world of certainties. And for the most part we like it this way. Many of these certainties serve us. We're pretty certain that the sun will rise each morning. We're certain that when we speak to someone they'll understand us. (Although people rarely perceive what we say exactly the way we mean it.) We're certain that we'll get up tomorrow morning. (Though we've seen there is no guarantee of this.) We're certain that we'll get from here to there without any incident.

Certainties can serve us. But they can also bind us. We can be certain that we won't get the job because we're not qualified enough. We can be certain that a relationship is too good to be true. (And if we're certain it's too good to be true, it will be too good to be true.) We can be certain that we won't be able to finish a race, but we're going to try. We can be certain that our lives are going to unfold the way we've been told, even though that way may not be how we would really like it to be.

Certainties can serve us, but the majority of the certainties we have are beliefs that are disempowering. They are beliefs which tie us to paradigms which don't allow for our growth, empowerment, and the full expression of ourselves. Most of the certainties which we hold onto are paradigms which keep us from reaching the life we desire or ought to be living, and stop us from Living in Vibrancy and experiencing the Glow of Being Alive.

I recently met a nurse who is what is referred to as a diploma nurse. She went through a three year training program to receive a nursing certificate. Another way to become a nurse is through a four year program that leads to a Bachelor's degree in nursing. The chief difference between the two paths is that the four year program has a much greater emphasis on administrative duties and statistics, things a typical clinical nurse will rarely ever use. In fact, the diploma nurse actually gets a much richer clinical experience during their training than a nurse who receives a Bachelor's degree, because much less time is spent on learning bureaucratic paper pushing. The diploma nurse comes out of their training better prepared to be a hands-on clinical nurse.

Now, one way is no better that the other. They are only different. However, in my friend's mind, she is certain that her degree is not as good as the other. She is certain that it is preferable to have the Bachelor's degree than the diploma certificate. This certainty prevents her from applying for certain jobs. Her certainty binds her to a particular paradigm and way of engaging the world, a way that is extremely disempowering. Her certainty keeps her bound to a place where in reality there are no bounds and an infinity of options.

Now you might comment and say, well, common knowledge of today's societal standards make it better to have the Bachelor's degree than the diploma. I would respond by saying that it is *her perceptions* and *her paradigms* that order *her reality*. The reality of the rest of the world doesn't matter. (And that's a certainty.) If her perception was that the diploma and her training is just as good as the Bachelor's degree, if not better by virtue of the much richer clinical experience she had, then her whole world would shift, and opportunities that she never imagined would open up for her. Our world is our world, and what the rest of the world does really doesn't matter. To change anything, we need to change *our world* by changing our perception of it first.

As we have seen previously, there are no guarantees about anything. In working with death, we realized that even though we believe and are certain we will be alive tomorrow, there's no guarantee. Likewise, we may be certain that we can't do or achieve something, but that certainty is also only a belief. There is no guarantee that we can't, although we tend to believe there is.

Mathematics supports this paradigm. This may seem like an odd construct, but it illustrates a very valid point. If I were to tell you that a group of ten monkeys given a large box of alphabet letters could assemble them into the complete works of Shakespeare, you'd say I was crazy. You'd say it was impossible. Yet mathematically there is a known, defined, statistical probability that it can happen. It's a very small probability, but it is a real, finite number. (However, as we'll see later, probabilities really don't matter.) It's not a certainty that it *cannot* happen. Actually, many scholars don't believe the works of Shakespeare were written by one person. They are *certain* that they are just too voluminous and perfect to have been created by one person. Why not? If it's possible that ten monkeys can do it, why not one man? Because we haven't experienced it personally and because we can't conceptualize it, we're *certain* it can't be. How we so severely limit ourselves!

Experience

Make a list of certainties in your life. You should list all of the things you are certain about, both bad and good. By bad and good I mean those things you are certain don't serve you any longer, (everything in our lives, even though we may now consider it bad, served us at some point), and those things that you are certain still do serve you. Include everything from, I'm certain my companion will be with me forever, and, I'm certain that I will stay in my job, to, I'm certain I won't get the promotion. Write down all of the certainties, those that serve you, and those that don't. This will be a long list because we uphold our world with certainties.

Now there are a number of ways to work with this list. The objective of all of them is to realize that we either create the certainties for ourselves, or we accept certainties we're given without reviewing and evaluating them ourselves. We need to realize that we order our world and our lives with the things we believe, but haven't proven to ourselves are certain. In truth, in our lives we're given a box of letters—what we do with them is up to us.

Start with the certainties which serve you, the ones you like and you want to hold onto. Examine them and see where they originated from. Have they come from your personal experience, or are they ideas you've accepted because someone gave them to you or because you want to believe in them? Are you certain you and your current companion will be together forever because you *know* it, or because you *believe* it? There is a difference. How can you know it for certain when forever hasn't arrived yet? It's all right to be certain of it, but know where the certainty originated from.

Next, work in the same manner with the certainties which don't serve you. Where have they come from? Are they things you know for certain, or are they ideas and beliefs you've accepted from family, peers, and the consensual world? Beliefs and certainties of the consensual are just that, beliefs. We can choose whether or not we want to subscribe to them. Are the certainties which don't serve you ideas you've examined and have consciously decided you desire to subscribe to, or are they concepts you've accepted as just the way things are because everyone else accepts them? Everything we hold for certain is a belief, nothing more. And what others believe and hold for certain doesn't have to be true for us. All that matters for us as individuals is what we choose to believe and hold for certain for ourselves and our world.

An alternate way to help realize where these ideas come from and how they affect us is to go through the list and give each item a number from one to ten, with ten being things that you are absolutely one hundred percent certain about, and one being things you are not really certain about. Now look at each item and understand why it received a particular number. Is the item a certainty because you've experienced it as such, or because you've been told it's that way and you accepted it as such? If you've experienced it as a certainty, maybe it's because you've chosen it as one by default, and now is the time to choose differently. If an item received a low number, ask yourself why? Find out why it's not for certain, and choose differently. It's your choice!

Holding

The interface between the First Circle, the Circle of Certainties, and the Second Circle, the Circle of Probabilities, is Holding. This means holding onto beliefs and ways of thinking that no longer serve us. It means retaining agreements and contracts which we've been given and accepted, but that we never consciously agreed to and never examined ourselves to see if we wanted to partake in them.

An example of one of these agreements is the way we're taught and expected to live our lives in the United States. We're taught to live the consensual paradigm: go to high school and then go to college, and then maybe graduate school, then get a job, work extremely hard until you're 65, then stop working, retire, and enjoy the golden years of your life. This is the typical paradigm we're taught by our media, advertising, and culture at large. It's how we're told we're supposed to live our lives. It's what we're supposed to do because we're told it's the best and it's the way everybody does it. It's not right or wrong. It's only one way. In India, one of the common paradigms is living through the four stages of life recognized there. They are youth, the householder, the elder, and the renunciate. In each stage the individual upholds certain societal duties. This paradigm is different than ours, and is neither right nor wrong. It is just one of the countless ways of living life.

Where did our consensual paradigm come from? I don't know! I really don't. I have some ideas, but it's not important where it came from. I do know that it works for some people. But I also know that for many people it falls flat and fails miserably. It's highly disempowering and for many people it leads to extreme regret for a life not lived to the fullest. It's an agreement many of us participate in by default and one that most of us never examine to see if it's the right one for us. There are many other paradigms we can live our lives by, and we can choose any of them. I'll give you one alternative.

Much of the paradigm we've just described, the consensual or normal, (and what's normal anyway but what the majority agrees to as what's right) is mixed up with our ideas of work and job–another paradigm which ought to be shifted. Part of my work with businesses is getting people to shift these paradigms. We're taught that our job and our work is a chore–a necessary evil we need to perform in order to make money. For many of us, our work becomes something we have to do when we would rather be doing something else. Even if we truly like what we do for a living, we sometimes fall prey to this idea and we allow our work to become less than satisfying. Work and money then get tied to the quest for material goods, another paradigm we've been given but many of us have not examined. We're not going to get into this one at the moment, but suffice to say the idea that more is better is something many of us never stop to examine.

Instead of our work being a job and a chore, an infinitely more empowering paradigm is that our work should be our craft, our passion. It should be one of those things that takes us into the timeless and that connects us to Source. Our work should be what we would rather be doing when we're doing something else. With this new perception of work, why would you want to stop doing it when you turn 65? If it's your passion, if it's what you do, why would you ever retire from it? Stories abound of South American medicine men and women who do ceremony and healing until well into their 80's and 90's. They *work* in the morning, and pass on (die) in the evening. There is one story in particular I remember of a shaman who performed a *Despacho*, a South American ceremony in which a ritual offering is made to the spirits, then passed on as he sat by the fire where he burned the offering. These people have followed their bliss. They have followed their calling and their passion until their time to pass on. It's very simple.

So an alternative paradigm to the way we're used to living in the world might be to not worry about what you're going to be doing when you're 65. You may not make it that far anyway. Be in your bliss, in the moment and on your path, and make your bliss what you do for your pay. Don't be concerned with amassing great fortunes for the security they will give you, or so that you can live off of them in your golden years after you retire to do all of the things you wished you could have done when you were younger but that you may not be able to do when you're older. Pace yourself. Enjoy each and every day. Each one is a gift of immense proportion. Love what you do and plan to be doing it when you pass on.

Our paradigms are our choice. We don't have to be part of the consensual ones by default. We don't have to hold on to any of them. Examine each and every paradigm, then choose those right for you. These paradigms are only agreements. We can make any agreement we desire and it will be binding until we decide to choose differently. Here is another alternative agreement of how we can order our lives.

I have an acquaintance, who when he was in his late teens, decided that every ten years he would change his occupation. He decided–he made a contract and agreement, a *mañay*, with himself–that no matter how successful he was at what he was doing, he would embark on something different. He's now in his sixties and he has had an incredible journey through life.

This man's journey goes directly against another life paradigm we're given, but that we never examine and therefore agree to by default. We're told, not necessarily directly, but forcefully nevertheless, that we have to pick one occupation and stay with it for life. This agreement goes against everything in the universe. Everything changes. We're the only beings that hate change so vehemently. If you go to school or receive training for a particular occupation and you love it, it's your bliss and you hold onto it for life, great. If you change and it becomes a chore, that's great too! Change it. Change what you do for your living. You haven't wasted any time. You haven't done anything bad or wrong. You've only changed, and change is natural. Change is the way of life.

Whoever said we have to pick one thing and stay with it for our whole life? I don't know! Probably *they* again. I do know that it's an agreement we all accept, and a contract we sign by default. I work with so many people who are changing, and who all complain about the time they've wasted doing what they've been doing. That's nonsense. Time is never wasted. Anything you do or have done is part of creating who you are.

Another belief and agreement that's wrapped up in this whole ball of yarn is that as you grow older you become too old to learn a new occupation. Again, that's nonsense. People do it all of the time. We are only as old, feeble, and untrainable as we think. If there's something you want to do you can do it. It's your choice. Follow your heart and negotiate your own agreements and contracts.

We've been given countless agreements and numerous contracts that we accept without consideration. Our ideas about money, status, material goods, joy and love, hope, religious faith, and the whole of how we order our lives are agreements we've been handed, but never examined to see if we would like to participate.

The single worst, most problematic and world threatening agreement we are given and accept as true is that our way, whether individually, societally, nationally, or culturally, is the best way. We in the United States are convinced that our way is the best way–period. And we spend an inordinate amount of time and resources trying to make other peoples live our way. We want everybody to be like us. To use an old euphemism: It's our way or the highway.

Our way is one way, and it's no better or worse than any other way. Our way has brought us incredible material prosperity but has left us void of depth and meaning, and has made much of the planet a wasteland because of our unbridled greed. Because we're taught and agree that our way is the only way, we become egocentric, ethnocentric, and nationalistic, and have no tolerance for any other way. How many wars have been fought over this premise? How many cultures along with their beauty and diversity have been lost because of this belief?

During the 1998 winter Olympics held in Japan, I happened to be in a restaurant while the opening ceremonies were being televised. The Sumo wrestlers were engaging in a show of their way, their ceremony and ritual. Now I know about Sumo wrestling. I used to practice a Japanese style of martial arts and have studied the Japanese traditions. Sumo is a beautiful way, an incredible art, and is highly respected and venerated in the Japanese culture. A woman in her late fifties was sitting at the table next to me. I overheard her commenting about how disgusting the wrestler was because he was so fat. And how she couldn't understand why he was the way he was, and didn't want to watch or look at him.

Her attitude is purely a result of agreements she's been given but never examined. Had she, and I mean her essence, her spirit or soul, been born in and taken form in Japan, she may have become the wife of a Sumo wrestler.

In my own medical training the same type of prejudice was present. We worked with residents from another training program. There were always arguments over whose way of doing a particular procedure was better. None of the ways were wrong, people just never examined why they were so adamant about their way. Was it because they examined their way themselves and came to their own agreements and conclusions? Or was it because they just accepted the agreements they were given? They were taught one way, and because it's the way they were taught and were told was right, it became the right way. It became the *only way*.

I recently met a man from the United States who works for the government. He spends the majority of his time in Bolivia. He was once told by his doctor, when requesting a routine physical exam before an extended trip to South America, that people shouldn't travel away from their home country. They should just stay home where they're supposed to be. This attitude of isolationism and fear of *the other* has caused us the majority of our problems throughout history.

Experience 1

Write down all of your beliefs. All of them. List every single belief you have about how the world is and operates, how you should live your life, and how you should engage the world. List every belief you have about yourself, your country, your family, your religion and about others–other families, religions, and cultures. This is going to be a long list. It needs to include everything. Every prejudice. Every agreement. Every thought and idea that orders your world.

Now, take a good look at them. How many of the things on the list have you really examined to see if you want them working in your life? How many have you consciously agreed to? And how many have you accepted by default? Which ones serve you now? Which ones do not serve you? How many prejudices have you accepted without any experience of them? Is the prejudice really *real*, or do you make it real in your life because you've been told to make it real? Remember, it's your life you're concerned with, not anyone else's. We are all responsible for only our own lives. And we get what we want. If we want a prejudice to be true in our lives, then it will. If we don't want it to be true in our lives, it won't be. How many opportunities have you missed because you have held onto a belief system which you never consciously chose? All of the things on your list are of your choosing. Every single one. And there's no reason in the world why you can't choose differently!

One of the best ways to convince yourself that these agreements are all relative is to learn about other cultures. Read about the Sumo tradition. Expose yourself to foreign countries and cultures. See that our way is not the only way. Yet we have to take this a step further, and this step is a very powerful one. It can be frightening because it breaks down all of the boundaries and barriers we create, consciously and unconsciously, to uphold our own, singular worlds and keep us as individuals separate from each other and *the other*.

Without understanding that beneath each unique way exists the same *being*, a person with the same hopes, fears, and desires, the same essence of beauty and divinity as you, exposing yourself to other cultures doesn't do any good. It's still you and them–*the other*–and they're different, and only one can be right. And you naturally prefer the right one to be you.

Experience 2

This next exercise should be done with someone from another culture, a culture as different from yours as you can imagine. If you don't know anybody that fits that bill, then make a new friend. Maybe someone else reading this book. Maybe someone at a meditation class, or any group that you may be involved in. If you aren't ready to, or can't find anybody that is very different from you, work with someone you know, but they should at least be a different religion or nationality. You need to do this experience with someone you consider different from you. The person should be like minded and also be looking for avenues of personal growth. Together you are going to do a meditation with all of the ritual and ceremony we've been talking about throughout this book. This meditation and exercise can also be done in a group and is excellent for use in a workshop setting.

Create a sacred space with all of the ritual you have learned to use so far. Create a space that is appropriate for a deep ceremony. Once the atmosphere is appropriate, sit facing your partner. You both should then soften your gaze and meditate into each other's eyes. Open yourself up. Become part of your partner's gaze and allow them to drift into yours. Don't be afraid to see. Don't be afraid of losing yourself. Let your energy, and your emotions flow freely.

What do you see deep in their eyes? What do you now believe about the old saying, "The eyes are the windows to the soul." In the past these words may have only been an agreement that you accepted. What are they now? Where has the other gone? There is old wisdom that says, "To see the face of God, look in a mirror." See the reflection of God in your partner's eyes, and know they are seeing the same reflection in yours.

Probabilities
The Second Circle

Many of the shamanic traditions believe that we have all selected how we are going to die. They believe we select our death, even before we are born. And this is true, both figuratively and literally. Our scientific studies and research data tell us that some percent of us are going to die of cancer. Some percent of us are going to die of heart disease. Some percent of us are going to die in an automobile collision. And so forth. We all live with the probabilities of certain things happening to us. There is a probability of living to an average age, and a probability of dying earlier or later than the average age. We have probabilities for everything. My mother had cancer, so the probability that I'll get it is X. The chances of me getting a certain job are Y. The probability that I'll_____, is_____. The list goes on forever.

Probabilities aren't always bad. They can also serve us. My plane probably won't crash. I'll probably come home from my trip safe. Because there's no history of cancer in my family, I'll probably be fine. We very frequently order our lives with probabilities, and it is certainly better than the certainties that we use to hold ourselves back. But we can do better. We can do much better.

207

Experience

What probabilities function in your life? Write them out. These should not be things you're certain about. These should be things that you believe can go any number of ways, and that you assign a chance or probability of them occurring one way or another. These can be anything. They can be medical probabilities as in the examples. Probabilities regarding a job, or a change of life situation. The probability of it raining on your picnic. Anything that you're not certain of which way it's going to turn out, but that you assign a probability.

Once you've got the items listed, work with them one by one. Where did that probability come from? Who put it there? Did it come from your family or peers? Did it come from the culture at large, or the eternally wise but unseen *they* we've talked about? Have you examined the probability yourself to see if it's one you want to agree to? Why have you colluded with the consensual and agreed to it if it doesn't serve you?

For illustration, let's work with an example from women's health which is very germane to our society, breast cancer. In general, statistics tell us that about one in ten women in the United States will develop breast cancer within their lives. (Some current data suggests that the number is now closer to one in three.) Now that's a probability, a statistic which relates to a whole population. But you are an individual woman, ***you are not the whole population***. You are you, and you create your own life and choices.

Now that statistic came from somewhere, and to discuss how we as a whole society chose that number would fill a book by itself. For now, let me point out that many scientists are coming to the conclusion, as we discussed in the first chapter regarding physics, that there is no pure subject–object relationship. No matter how much we delude ourselves into believing so, there is absolutely no such thing as an unbiased observation or a blind study. There can be no perception of anything without an interaction between the observer and the observed, and that interaction, the act of observing, affects what is being observed. We select outcomes. We choose outcomes. And in the same way we choose as individuals, we can choose as a group. And as a group we have chosen that one out of ten number.

We've seen this working in our world dramatically in what has been called the Hundredth Monkey Effect. In brief, it was observed in an isolated population of monkeys, that once a critical number of the population learned a certain task, members who had no contact with those who were originally doing the task began performing it. They seemed to have learned by magic. And further, monkeys in populations geographically isolated from the first population also began performing the task as a group. This implies that once a critical number of members of a group learn or believe something, it rapidly becomes an attribute and truth for the whole group.

Despite our popular wisdom, we aren't that much different than monkeys. Once someone believes in a certain number, and then convinces others to believe in that number as a truth, it rapidly becomes a truth for the whole population. This happens in our reality all of the time.

Now, back to the statistic regarding breast cancer. We can work with the number in a few ways. First, a one out of ten chance of developing breast cancer seems like a high number. And actually, it is high. If you had a one out of ten chance of winning a million dollar lottery, you'd be mortgaging your house to buy tickets. But a nine out of ten chance of not developing breast cancer is higher. A ninety percent chance of not choosing a life-threatening disease is great! It's the old half-full or half-empty glass metaphor. If you choose to engage the world in a half-empty way, then you get a half-empty world. If you choose to engage the world in a half-full manner, you get a half-full world. (But why not engage the world and life in a completely full manner? More about this later.) Don't dwell on the outcomes that you don't want. Focus on the outcomes that you prefer. It's your choice. Where you put your energy and your intent should be on what you desire, not on what you're worried about happening. Why worry about a one out of ten probability when the nine out of ten is much higher?!

Second, you are an individual. You are not the whole system. The probabilities apply to the whole, not to the separate parts. This can be a tough concept to grasp. All of the great mystics and sages speak of a universal oneness, connectedness, and sameness. At the same time, each of them also speaks of an individuality and uniqueness. A sage simultaneously sees the oneness of all there is and the uniqueness of everything. The sages are aware that each human being is a manifestation of the one Divine Energy, but that at the same time, each person presents unique potential.

Now how do we make sense of that? We don't. We can't. We have no way to fit that concept into the rational framework and syntax through which we view ourselves and the world. We don't make sense of it, we experience it! We experience it through working The Steps to Vibrancy, being in the Empty Space, or engaging in any meditation system that works for us. We experience it, then we use that experience and knowledge to transform our lives.

You are equally as much an individual as a part of the whole. Being an individual means not having to be part of the consensual. Being an individual means having the ability to choose. It means choosing what you want, and how you want to perceive and engage the world, yourself, and any disease. Do you want to be the one out of ten, or do you want to be one of the nine out of ten? Choose even further. Choose to be one of the ten out of ten that aren't afflicted with the disease. Choose a probability of zero for yourself. Choose for yourself. Anything is possible, and we'll see this is so in the Third Circle.

Probabilities are just that, probabilities. They are possibilities given a number, nothing more. It's how we perceive them and how we view them that makes them real for us or not. The energy we give them is what makes them bear on our lives. When we change our perception, we change our world. And how we perceive the world is up to us. It's our choice!

Choice, Possibilities, & Creation

The Third Circle is the Realm of Possibilities. It's beyond probabilities. And it's so far beyond certainties that a circle is closed. It's a place where there are no certainties, yet, everything is for certain because anything and everything can happen. Any and all possibilities exist, anything can be for certain, and it's simply a matter of our choice. The interface between the Second Circle and the Third Circle is Choice. We can choose. We can choose any possibility we want. That's the whole theme of The Steps to Vibrancy. We can make the choice to step out of the consensual world, step through the first two circles, and step into the Third Circle, a place where it's entirely up to us to choose and create.

Consider any current situation in your life–any situation. Make a list of all of the possibilities. I mean every single one of the possibilities which can occur in that particular situation. All of them. Every single one. Include every one that you would like to see happen, and every one that you would like not to occur. List every single possibility, no matter how outrageous it may seem to you. From winning the lotto to dying tomorrow, include every possible outcome you can envision.

Now look at the list and pick one of the possibilities. That's right, pick the one you want to occur. It's that simple. Choose one. Be certain it's the one you really want though. (We in fact always get what we want, we just don't realize that we're choosing it.) In the realm of the Third Circle anything is possible, and each possibility is equally possible. This warrants repeating: *Each possibility is equally possible*. There are no odds or probabilities as we're used to considering. Once we've stepped out of the consensual world which tells us what's for certain and what's probable, everything is equally possible. It's really just that simple. We live within eternity although we don't realize it, and we certainly don't know how to utilize it. In eternity everything is equally possible. Everything.

The Third Circle is the realm of eternity. That is, eternity manifest in time and space. Each and every moment is an eternity unto itself. But how do we utilize this fact? How do we even comprehend it?

First, by experiencing, knowing, and embodying the first four Steps to Vibrancy: Take Responsibility, Get Into Your Power, Eliminate Excuses, and Step Into The Empty Space. Second, by understanding the Circles of Emergence, and understanding that the world we've been given and live in, a world of defined probabilities and certainties, is only one world, and we can live in whatever world we choose. And third, by then bringing back our choice from the Empty Space. Yes–Now we get to utilize our connection to the Empty Space.

Beyond the Third Circle is the Empty Space. It's the place of the timeless, eternity within eternity. It's Source, the oneness that we're all part of, the Void where everything exists. Between the Third Circle and the Empty Space is Creation. Within the Third Circle, we choose our possibilities, then we enter the Empty Space with that choice. Upon returning to the Third Circle we create. We bring eternity into our world of time and space. It's really that simple.

The not so simple part is two-fold. (There's always a catch, isn't there!) First, convincing ourselves we are creative beings and can do it. And second, releasing the conflicts, agreements, and consensual programming that prevent us from choosing, from really making a choice at a cellular, bodily, mental, and spiritual, I'm **one hundred percent** certain of that choice, level. The Steps to Vibrancy lead us to overcoming these not so simple parts. So how do we really do this?

When we're in the Empty Space we have no thoughts. Our ego identity, what we identify with as ourselves dissolves completely, and what remains is the pure Source, the pure creative potential that is our essence. This essence is beyond anything we can ever categorize or conceptualize ourselves as. With the ego dissolved, all conflicts, agreements, and consensual programming are gone. There is only Source, the pure, single, unadulterated potential for creation. A single thought, a single focused thought where it is the only thought occurring is an act of creation. This thought is planting a seed in the rich, fertile soil of the Empty Space. It is a pure, unopposed focus of our attention and intent, and that's the critical part. The key is an unopposed focus of our attention and intent, and that happens within the Empty Space.

We've used the word intent before. Intent is one of those things that can be known, but is difficult to describe and talk about. Intent is a focus of will or thought. Unopposed intent is when the attention is fully on one thought. Unopposed intent is where our attention is consumed by only one thought. It's where the totality of our being is held by a single, simple, purposeful act of creation. The single thought is the only thought, it is the only thing occupying the totality of consciousness. Unopposed intent is where one and only one thought has the totality of our attention, or to put it the other way, the totality of our attention is occupied by one and only one thought. When we're in the Empty Space, this single thought becomes our act of creation. That's why the Empty Space is so important. It's the place we choose from. It's the place where we make our choice, then we create and manifest it by returning to the Third Circle, the realm of possibilities. So, let's give it a try!

Experience

Make a choice about something in your life that you want to see occur. Start with something simple, something that doesn't have a lot of baggage attached to it. By this I mean something that isn't, at least as far as you can tell, tied up with a lot of other issues that need to be released through the other Steps to Vibrancy. It can be as simple as deciding that you will hear from an old friend who you haven't spoken to in a while. Or resolving a disagreement with a companion or acquaintance. Or manifesting that a particular situation will resolve in your favor. Pick the situation and choose specifically what you would like to have happen. You need to be focused and specific on the outcome. Be very specific, because you will get what you ask for.

Next, go into the private, sacred space you have created for yourself. Light a candle, burn some incense, do whatever you want to make the space different from the outside world. I recently spoke to a healing group where the leader used a small energy chime at the beginning of the meeting. As we began she announced that at the sound of the chime the world we had spent the day in was to be left behind, and with the sound we would be in a sacred space where miracles are commonplace. She sounded the chime and the room we were in became different. I can't rationally describe the difference, but it changed. We had all stepped into a different reality. Do whatever it takes to transport yourself into a sacred space.

Play your music or drumming, or sit in silence, whatever helps you to connect with the Empty Space. Then leave. Leave yourself and your world. Leave all of the constraints you've been given and all of the agreements you've been handed and accepted but never consciously agreed to. Leave the world of the consensual and step into the Empty Space. Go to the place of no thought where anything and everything exists. Step into the Empty Space with the intent of bringing back with you the desire you have chosen. Go to the Empty Space clear, pure, and with only the intent of manifesting your choice within the field of time and space.

Once you're in the Empty Space bask in it. Float in the joy, comfort, and easeful repose of eternity where there are no distinctions between you and anything else because *you are everything*. There is no *other* in the Empty Space. There is only Source, and you and Source are indistinguishable. Enjoy the splendor and magnificence of the Empty Space. Experience the wholeness and perfection of your own beautiful uniqueness within the backdrop of eternal oneness and completion. Just be, and when you are ready, create.

Once you're free of all of the encumbrances you've been given by life, and when you have no thoughts, bring the one single thought of what you are going to create into focus. Bring that single thought, and only that thought into being. Become that thought. Be it. See yourself as it. Feel the emotion behind the beingness of whatever it is that you desire to become, or manifest. This is much easier to do than it sounds because, in fact, you already are it. Within the Empty Space you are everything. Within the Empty Space there is no separateness, and there is no *other*. See whatever it is that you *already are* manifesting within your life, within the field of time and space. See it happening with your vision, and see it happening within your heart. Feel it within the totality of your being so completely that there's no room in your vision or being for anything else except that one eternal moment.

This is much more than a visualization. This is an act of creation because it's occurring from a place of stillness. It's occurring from a place of oneness with the creative Source of which we are all a part. Visualizations are marvelous tools, that's why we use them, but the only way any of them work is when they happen within, and out of, a place of complete stillness where there are no other opposing, conflicting, or distracting images. And when we are empty, in the Empty Space, we are in the realm of stillness and oneness that is the creative Source of everything.

See, and feel, what you are creating. Feel and see your unique creation within the stillness of yourself, and then project it out into the stillness of the Empty Space. Hold the image and feeling within your heart, then send out the order to create like a beam of light projecting out from your essence into the eternity of the Void. See this beam of the light of your vision, of your focused intent, exploding like a new galaxy bursting into creation for the first time. Feel it filling the totality of yourself and your consciousness. See and feel the vision of your creation wrapping around you as you become it, and it becomes you.

While you're in the Empty Space allow the image and feeling of your creation to burst forth from the totality of who you are. Continually feel the laser-like, focused attention and intent emanating from your heart, your Source, and melding with the infinite and eternal Source that is indistinguishable from your own. Bask and float, now and forever, within the eternity of the moment of your creation.

Once you've finished in the Empty Space, return to the Third Circle, it's your home within the field of time and space. There's no reason to go into any of the other circles. The object is to live within the Third Circle where anything and everything is possible, *and is equally probable*. As you cross back into the Third Circle from the Empty Space you cross the threshold of creation. You engage as a complete and total partner with Source in creating your world. Cross the threshold of creation and bring the gift of your vision into the world you have created for yourself within the field of time and space.

Back in your own world, and your personal sacred space, spend some time feeling your body. Within the Empty Space you have separated from your body. Now, once you've returned, feel within your body the reality of your vision and the taste of your creation. Feel, viscerally, what it is like to be the you that you have created within the Empty Space and have now brought back into your world of time and space. What is the bodily sensation associated with the gift you've given yourself? Where does it live within your body? Feel the emotion behind the creation you have just manifested and cement it into your body and your world.

As you settle in and become more grounded within the here and now, again, feel the force of your creation extending outward from your heart, your source, and enveloping the totality of your world. Feel your world shifting as the power of your act of creation comes to manifest within the field of time and space. Let the vision of your creation percolate through the luminous fibers of your being and your world.

Once you've become proficient at entering the Empty Space and planting the message of creation, one trip will be enough. In fact, Living in Vibrancy is living with one foot in the Empty Space and one foot in the Third Circle. (More about this in the next chapter.) In the beginning, while you're a novice, take the journey you've just been on at least three times a week. As many times as you can is best, and this can mean two or three times a day. It takes some practice to be able to enter the Empty Space completely free and empty, and hold one single, unopposed thought of creation. So do the journey as much as you can. It's that simple. Really.

During the times when you are not *officially* Stepping into The Empty Space as a formal exercise, you should be holding the thought of your creation. Again, the goal of Living in Vibrancy is to walk the edge of Creation between the Third Circle and the Empty Space, and to flick in and out of the Empty Space like an incandescent light flicks on and off. For now, as you walk within your world of time and space, know that you are creating it every second. Know that every single thing you do and every single thought you have is an act of creation, and hold the vision of your creation, what you placed into the Empty Space, with you at all times. Feel and see yourself in that vision with every breath that you take. And as you walk with beauty and the knowledge and vision of your creation held dearly, be aware of the world around you. Become aware of the synchonicities and serendipities that are ushering your creation into your life. Take a step back from trying to micromanage every detail and *allow* your creation to manifest. The universe is very accommodating, and will accommodate itself to whatever you create. This can be as blatant as something manifesting right before your eyes–water into wine–or more subtle. It's entirely up to us what we wish to create. And it is up to us–**it's our choice**–what agreements and contracts we wish to keep and which ones we desire to void.

I used to tell people that it would be much simpler if the universe would just talk to us in a very simple form, like a billboard with huge black and white lettering answering whatever question we've asked. I used to say that the universe speaks to us in metaphors and clues and just doesn't give us the clear, black and white messages we would like. I don't say that anymore. A while ago I was leading a weekend workshop. One of the gentlemen was working with the energy of a turtle–his totem animal–all day on Saturday. We did a ceremony Saturday evening and he drove home. He arrived early Sunday morning very excited. His enthusiasm was palpable and contagious. "Richard," he said loudly as he came up to me. "Richard, you won't believe it. I was driving home last night and I looked up, and there, right in front of me was this huge billboard with a turtle on it. I couldn't believe it. I pulled over, looked out the window, and nodded my head. Wow, what an affirmation!"

Yes, what an affirmation! I eventually saw the billboard also. It was a huge red sign with a turtle on it. That's all there was on the sign, just this gigantic turtle. Underneath the turtle was written, "I brake for turtles." It was more than eye catching. You couldn't miss it, and you couldn't figure out what it meant. The sign was only up for about a month, and turned out to be a prelude to an advertising campaign for a new ice cream flavor. The important point is that it was up at just the right time for my friend to experience the synchronicity and affirmation he needed for the work he was doing.

The universe speaks to us every moment. We just need to be open and aware. All we need to do once we've planted the seed of creation in the Empty Space is allow our creation to manifest within the world of time and space. It's that simple.

Once you've experienced creation with simple things, move along. We create the totality of our world. Everything. *Every thing.* This is a tough concept to grasp, but it's true. There is nothing that we can't change, absolutely nothing, because everything, every circumstance and situation in our lives is our creation. Since we have created everything, there is nothing that we can't change. There is absolutely nothing within our lives that we do not have control over. Absolutely nothing. Once you've created on a smaller level, one that is easy for you to accept, then move along. Move up to those big things that always seemed out of your control. Take responsibility for what you have created, because you have created everything. Then change whatever you want. Create something new. Create the life you desire and Live in Vibrancy. It's your choice, and only yours. Choose.

Vibrancy

The Glow of Being Alive

One of the signs of a life well lived is the amount of sunrises and sunsets you participate in.

Marie Reilly

WE'VE ARRIVED. WE'VE REACHED THE LAST STEP. We've Taken Responsibility. We've found, and Gotten Into Our Power. We've Eliminated Excuses. We've Stepped Into The Empty Space. And we've Chosen Our Circle. Now we're at the last step, *Vibrancy: The Glow of Being Alive*. Actually, we've been here all along, and Vibrancy isn't really a step. It's a state of being. And it's a state of being we've lived in since our birth. The problem is we haven't been taught this. We've been conditioned and made to believe that Vibrancy is something we have to search for and arrive at. We've been told that it's something outside of ourselves, and like revelation, bliss, and salvation we have to wait for some predetermined time in the future for it to come to us. There is no waiting. It's here, around all of us, right now. We're in it, and we're in it all of the time. We just don't realize it. We live in the garden. We've never been cast out. And when we change our perception of the world, that's when the world changes. It's a pretty heady proposition, but it's true, and Living The Steps to Vibrancy will forever change your perception of the world.

Last year I worked with a woman in her late thirties. She has been searching all of her life for her personal connection to the transcendent. The indigenous medicine traditions were new to her, but she had gone through just about every other type of spiritual discipline. During the conversation we had as part of her healing, one of the comments she made was that she knows intellectually that the transcendent, the divine, the godhead is within her. She emphatically pointed to her chest as she said, "I know it's here." She made similar statements a number of times during our talk. Then, as our conversation continued, she commented on how frustrated she was because she couldn't find the Source. She told me, "I can't bring it into myself."

I pointed out to her that, yes, she knows at an intellectual level what she's been taught, but she has never embodied it. She has never felt or truly owned the teachings. She can state that she knows the divine is within, but when she speaks freely without forethought the residual programming within her comes out. Intellectually she knows the divine is within, yet she says, "I can't bring it *into* myself." Unconsciously, and we know that the unconscious is anything but unconscious, she still accepts the propositions she's been given, namely, that the divine is outside of her. As I pointed this out to her, she had an "Ah-ha" realization which showed her that she still has some work to do Taking Responsibility and releasing the old agreements she was handed.

Our conversation also turned to the Void, or what we've called the Empty Space, the Source of everything. The question came up as to just where the Empty Space is located. We tend to think that we're here, and that the Empty Space is *out there* somewhere. (We've talked about this before in reference to the night sky.) We have a concept of space and distance in which we define two points, then we have to be at one or the other, and have to travel a set distance from one to the other. Well, that's only our perception. It's the only perception we know. It's the only one we've been given, it's the only one we can understand, and it's the only one we can accept.

Well space, just like time, has many facets. There is a realm where space, just like time, is not like we think it is. Just as we can exist in an eternal moment of now by stepping outside of the linear time we're used to, we can exist in an eternal place of here. This is a place where there is no *here* or *there*. It's where there is no distance from point "a" to point "b." Everything just is, and is all at once. It's all *here*, because there is no *there*. This is the Void. This is the Empty Space. It's the place where creation springs forth and rushes like a blast of wind into our world of linear time and space.

The point of all of this is that the Empty Space is not *out there* somewhere. We don't leave where we are physically and go somewhere else to be in the Empty Space. **The Empty Space, the Void, the Source, is right here. We're in it!** We're in it right now, this singular, very precious moment. We exist within the Source. We exist in the place of creativity. In fact, we are it! We are the creative principle, each and every one of us, and we create with every thought, every word, every emotion. The Void is all around us, and we don't see it. Remember, "The kingdom is spread upon the earth, and men do not see it," and, "...the life is the light of man. And the light shines in darkness: and the darkness comprehends it not." We don't see it for many reasons, the primary one being that since our birth we have been conditioned to collude with the consensual and accept the consensual definition of reality. And that definition includes the proposition that we are at the mercy of forces outside of ourselves. Once the consensual becomes part of our operating system and way of engaging the world and our lives, it's the way we live, and it produces the world we live in. The consensual becomes our view of the world and we give away our true power and potential.

A dear friend of mine and I have had an ongoing discussion about the nature of the universe. The question we debated was whether the nature and essence of the universe is hostile and predatory, or kind and loving. The universe is neither. Both of those views are judgments and perceptions. **The universe is accommodating**. It accommodates itself to whatever our idea and perception of it is. If our idea is that it's predatory, then it's predatory. If our idea is that it's kind and loving, then it's kind and loving. The universe is anything we want it to be because it's our creation. We are in the Empty Space right now, in this eternal moment of now, and creating as we go. We're writing the script of our lives and of our worlds in just the same way as these words are flowing onto the screen in front of me.

So, what is Living in Vibrancy? We are Living in Vibrancy right now. *We are* the Creative Principle manifest in time and space. It's not out there somewhere, it's right here within ourselves. Living in Vibrancy means recognizing that the world is our creation, and realizing this fact on not only a superficial level, but on a deep, visceral level with the totality of our being. Our thoughts uphold the world, and when we change our thoughts about the world, the world changes. It's simply a matter of choice. And it's our choice. We only have to choose.

Living in Vibrancy means knowing that the world is our creation and loving it as such. It means loving the world, everything in the world, the same as we might love a newborn son or daughter. It's the love of creator for creation, whatever form that creation takes. It means loving ourselves completely, totally, and unconditionally because we are also our creation. We have each created the self that we are. And before we even consider changing who we are, we need to own and take responsibility for who we are, because we created the man or woman reading these words. Then we need to love ourselves with that same unconditional love we have for anything we have created.

Living in Vibrancy means acknowledging life for its raw, uncensored beauty which transcends all of our judgments and ideas of right doing and wrong doing. Living in Vibrancy means counting the number of sunrises and sunsets you participate in. Sit with a sunrise or sunset and feel within yourself the emotions that are stirred from out of the deep, dark, still pool of your being. These emotions are a guide, a link, a luminous thread to the creative power that you have. Feel these emotions. Feel these things that go beyond words, these things you can know but not speak about, then carry them with you as you walk through your life. Hold them as a dictionary as you write the screenplay of your life's drama as you're playing the leading role.

We sometimes talk about the medicine people, the shamans, sages, and seers, as living with one foot in both worlds. They have one foot in the Empty Space, and one foot in the field of time and space at all times. They shuttle their attention, focus, and awareness back and forth. They are constantly creating their reality with every single thought and action.

The idea of going back and forth to the Empty Space is attractive because it helps our rational self to comprehend something which is difficult for it to understand. But Living in Vibrancy is not a bouncing back and forth between two worlds. It means *being in*, and *living in* a state of transcendence *all of the time*. It means living in the garden. It means recognizing that we are in the Empty Space and what we do with it is entirely and completely up to us. It means knowing and expressing the idea that we can live exactly and however we chose. It means, as one shaman says, cresting all of the time. We have complete choice and freedom to create the lives and world that we desire, and Living in Vibrancy means living in the glow and balance of that knowledge.

Living in Vibrancy is not some far off goal, or some secret, esoteric knowledge that necessarily takes a lifetime cloistered in an ashram to gain. There are no secret codes or handshakes to gain entry. Living in Vibrancy is sacred, and sacred is not secret. Living in Vibrancy is living in the here and now, recognizing the vibrancy, the energy, the glow of the moment, and creating the next moment however we choose, unencumbered by the social conditioning and agreements we've been handed. It means taking hold of the Divinity that we each are, not relinquishing that power to anyone or any institution, and letting it shine into the world of our creation. It's totally, completely, entirely our choice. Go ahead–Choose.

Living In Vibrancy

We have been through The Steps to Vibrancy. The Steps, simply put, lead us to the power we all have within ourselves, but that we've given up. The Steps take us directly to the divinity within. For some people, one time through The Steps may take you to the place of understanding that we have commonly called enlightenment. For others, it may take a number of times walking The Steps. For most, Living The Steps will be an ongoing process you engage in every day. Whatever they are or become for you is all right. The point is to use them. Use them and *live them*.

In the beginning of this book we discussed many of the spiritual traditions and made the analogy of these traditions to spokes on a wheel, with all of the spokes leading to the grand "Truth" in the middle. Many people *spirit shop* and engage this tradition this week, and another one the next week, because one practice or another didn't work. **They all work**. They all lead to "Truth." But for a practice to work, **it has to be lived**. And to live a practice means just that, **live the practice–walk your talk**. It means giving up all of your old thoughts, ideas, and concepts about the way the world is or should be, and engaging the world in a completely different manner. But this giving up can be difficult, because it means giving up everything you thought was real and unchanging. It means giving up the you who you think you are, and this can be frightening. To Live The Steps to Vibrancy means to *live them*. And if you live them, they will work.

Once the Steps are embodied you arrive at a place of Vibrancy, and a Glow of Aliveness filters from you into the world surrounding you. As you shift, so does your world. Below are some ways to maintain this shift and *Live in Vibrancy*.

Stay in balance

When you are in balance, your world is in balance. Maintain your equilibrium no matter what the situation. As you learn to walk in balance, the situations that test your balance will become fewer and fewer.

Hold the feeling

Vibrancy is a feeling. It's a mood. It's a sensation beyond words. You've experienced it when you were in the Empty Space. You've experienced it when living in your power. Hold onto that feeling and mood at all times.

Walk in beauty

The universe is accommodating. If you expect ugliness, that's what you will get. If you walk in beauty, beauty will return to you a thousand-fold.

See the beauty in all things

All things are creation. Everything and everyone is not only connected, but all made of the same *stuff*. It's all part of the transcendent. See the remarkable beauty of all things in your daily life.

Expect what you want

If you desire something, truly desire it and desire to create it, expect it. All of the talk about not holding onto expectations is a paradigm—one you can choose, or not choose. How can you expect to get something if you don't expect it? You can create anything that you desire. Anything. So you should expect it. And you will get it providing all of the underlying conflicts, and there can be many, have been released.

Practice non-judgment

Do not judge yourself, and especially do not judge others. See actions and events for what they are, actions and events—nothing more. They are not good or bad. If you do not like a situation, take responsibility for it, understand why you chose it, then release it and choose differently. But whatever the situation, never, never, pass judgment on it.

Stay out of other people's dramas

Be compassionate and empathic, but don't get caught up in other people's lives. They make their own choices. Let them. When they are ready, they will choose differently. Just listen, and *be* for the other person without judgment or giving advice. It is the finest gift one can give another. This is known as compassion.

Speak your truth, always

We've seen how powerful words are. Always, always, always speak your truth, from your heart. Everybody speaks about loving yourself. The best way to do that is to be yourself, and the best way to be yourself is to always speak your truth, from your heart.

No colluding with the consensual

Be you, whatever that means to you. Period. You are the only person you are beholden to, and you do not have to be part of the consensual.

Look into other people's eyes

Look into the eyes of other people when you talk to them. It will quickly cut through everything and get to the level where the essence of what is truly important is brought to the surface.

See yourself in others

The Buddha said, "See yourself in others, then whom can you hurt? What harm can you do?" This is self-explanatory.

Don't cling

Don't cling to anything. When you don't cling, you aren't attached. When you aren't attached, you have nothing to lose. When you have nothing to lose, you are free. When you are free, you have everything to gain.

Don't know

Don't know. Don't know how something is going to happen. Just know it will happen. When you don't know, you leave room for magic, and magic is all around us. In fact, we are the magic.

Know

Know that you are the creative force in your own life. You are your own Source. *You are the magic!*

Let go of the trapeze

Let go of the trapeze of the consensual and of the security of the known. Let go even if you can't see the net. Another trapeze will always come. Remember, no back doors.

Stop understanding

Stop trying to understand everything. You can't. And you don't have to. Take the energy expended in trying to understand and use it to create. Use it to *be* and experience joy.

Spend time in nature

Spend time in the woods or at the beach or lake. It's going home. It's a place of balance. And it's where the still voice inside is not overshadowed by the voices of people and the consensual understanding.

Listen

Listen to the soft voice within. Hear it, listen to it, and learn to trust it.

Don't be surprised

Don't be surprised when magic happens. It's the norm, not the extraordinary. Miracles happen every day, yet there really are no miracles. There are just those things that don't fit in with the consensual understanding of things.

Live in your own world, and let others live in theirs

When we talk about children we frequently refer to them, "Living in their own world." They are just fine in their own worlds until we force them to be part of ours. Children know. They know those things we search for. Live in whatever world you want. It's simply a choice. And let other people live in whatever world they desire.

When others judge you, let them be

Let other people have their say, and then smile, thank them, and live your life. Don't get caught up in their beliefs and prejudices. See what is talking. Is it their pride, or their ignorance, or their upbringing?

Don't try to change anybody

Leave others to have their own experiences. If and when they want to change, they will. It's only your job to save the world if you choose it to be.

Fear not

When you've met death, and have given up clinging, what is there to fear? Nothing!

Have knowledge, not hope

Hope is as great of an enemy as fear. Don't have hope, have knowledge.

Don't worry, be happy

Happiness is purely a state of mind. And it works. What else is there to say?

Watch your moods

We tend to think that situations determine our moods. However, it's our moods that call the situations into our lives. Strive to keep your mood one that fosters who you want to be.

Poetry

Life is poetry. Life is a poem. See it as such. Write it out. Write the poem of your life.

Live in the sacred

There is no difference between sacred and secular. Everything is sacred. And sacred is not secret. Engage the world as such and let the world see who you are.

Work with the energy

Engage events and situations at the most basic level, the energetic. This is how creation occurs.

Walk in the dark

At night, in the dark, it's easier to create than in the day. It's easier to create something new out of the darkness of the Void than to change what's already been made that fits in with the consensual. It's all right to be in the dark. In the dark everything is formless. Out of the dark we can create any form we desire.

Time out is not time lost

Spend time with yourself. Spend time alone, not doing anything. It's the best time you can spend. It's when the real knowing takes place. It's when we hear the whisper of who we are.

Allow

Allow those things you desire to flow into your life. Get out of the way and allow them to occur.

Trust

Trust, unlike fear and hope can be a double-edged sword. Trust linked with the hope that something will come to pass will sink you every time. Trust linked with the *knowledge* that you can, and in fact *do create your own reality*, is a direct link to the singular source of creation we all are.

Living in Vibrancy is not some far off, improbable or impossible goal. It's not secret knowledge reserved for a mystic on a mountain top, or a holy person or saint. Living in Vibrancy and experiencing the life you ought to be living is right here, right now. The peace, wholeness, knowingness, and creative potential of the Christ Light, or the Buddha Consciousness, or the Divine Energy, is available to each and every one of us in this singular, precious moment we call our life.

The life you ought to be living is waiting for you this second. It's stalking you just as you are seeking it. It's only a matter of choice. Go ahead. Choose. It's that simple. It truly is that simple. And, it's up to you. It's your choice!

235

AUTHOR'S NOTE

Native people across the globe all recognize the importance of community when venturing into the unknown to seek healing and their own becoming. This sense of community is especially important when you live in consensual world which does not honor those who choose to become who they want to be.

To this end I humbly request your short stories of how The Steps to Vibrancy, or being on any spiritual path, has transformed your life into the one you want it to be. These stories, the poetry of your life, may be published in a forth coming book or in the *Cholla Wayra*–Winds of Vision–newsletter.

To submit a story, or be put on the newsletter mailing list, please contact me at the address below.

With warmth and love,

Richard

Dr. Richard Sandore
c/o Rikuys Press
Post Office Box 540
Wadsworth, Illinois 60083
shaman@enteract.com
www.soaringspirit.com

BIBLIOGRAPHY & PERMISSIONS

Abrams, David. *The Spell of The Sensuous: Perception and Language in a More Than Human World.* New York: Pantheon Books, 1996. Selections reprinted with permission. All rights reserved.

Arnold, Edwin., ed. *The Bhagavad Gita.* California: World Library Inc., 1991.

Barks, Coleman., ed. *The Essential Rumi.* New York: HarperCollins, 1995. Selections reprinted with permission. All rights reserved.

Campbell, Joseph. *Transformations of Myth Through Time.* New York: Harper & Row, 1990. Selections reprinted with permission. All rights reserved.

Capra, Fritjof. *The Tao of Physics.* New York: Bantam, 1984.

Carus, Paul., ed. *Buddha: His Life and Teachings.* California: World Library Inc., 1991.

Castaneda, Carlos. *Tales of Power.* New York: Simon & Schuster, 1974. Selections reprinted with permission. All rights reserved.

Confucius. *Confucian Analects.* California: World Library Inc., 1991.

Cumes, Carol & Valencia, Romulo Lizarrago. *Pachamama's Children.* Minnesota: Llewellyn Publications, 1995. Selections reprinted with permission. All rights reserved.

Dossey, Larry. *Healing Words: The Power of Prayer and the Practice of Medicine.* New York: HarperCollins, 1994.

Goswami, Amit. *The Self-Aware Universe: How Consciousness Creates the Material World.* New York: Putnam, 1995.

Hagerbaumer, Jim. *Hallelujah.* Unpublished poetry, 1998. Reprinted with permission. All rights reserved.

Halifax, Joan. *Shamanic Voices: A Survey of Visionary Narratives*. New York: E. P. Dutton, 1979

Horan, Paula. *Empowerment through Reiki*. Wisconsin: Lotus Light Publications, 1996.

Kharitidi, Olga. *Entering The Circle: Ancient Secrets of Siberian Wisdom Discovered by a Russian Psychiatrist*. New York: HarperCollins, 1997. Selections reprinted with permission. All rights reserved.

Muller, Max., ed. *The Upanisads*. New York: Dover, 1962.

Narby, Jeremy. *The Cosmic Serpent*. New York: Putnam, 1998.

Nayanatiloka, ed. *The Word of Buddha*. California: World Library Inc., 1991.

Osbon, Diane K., ed. *Reflections on the Art of Living: A Joseph Campbell Companion*. New York: HarperCollins, 1991. Selections reprinted with permission. All rights reserved.

Perkins, John. *Shapeshifting: Shamanic Techniques for Global and Personal Transformation*. Vermont: Destiny Books, 1997. Selections reprinted with permission. All rights reserved.

Perkins, John. *The World Is As You Dream It: Shamanic Teachings From The Amazon And Andes*. Vermont: Destiny Books, 1994.

Robinson, James M., ed. *The Nag Hammadi Library*. New York: Harper-Collins, 1990. Selections reprinted with permission. All rights reserved.

Suares, Carlo. *The Cipher of Genesis*. Maine: Weiser, 1992. Selections reprinted with permission. All rights reserved.

Thomas Nelson, Inc. *The Holy Bible, New King James Version*. National Publishing Company, 1985.

Webster's New Universal Unabridged Dictionary. New Jersey: Barnes & Noble Books, 1994.

Doctor Richard Sandore is a Western trained physician who practiced Obstetrics for nine years. During this time he came to know the indigenous medicine traditions which taught him the difference between healing and curing, and a path to true healing.

He now has a healing practice north of Chicago, lectures, writes, teaches spirituality and empowerment based on the native medicine traditions, works with business and the concept of spirit in the workplace, and leads healing journeys across the world.